Dermatology Multiple Choice Questions & Notes

For Medical Students and General Practitioners

By Abigail Johnston

Mostafa Khalil

Bridging the Gap Academy

Copyright © 2021 Abigail Johnston & Mostafa Khalil

All rights reserved.

ISBN: 9798592701849

Dedication

We dedicate this book to our family, who have been very supportive and have encouraged and inspired us throughout the entire process. Thank you, Dr Mohamed Khalil and Dr Sahar Hussein. Thank you, Lesley Johnston, Jim Johnston, Maureen Smith and Alec Johnston.

Table of Contents

Table of Contents 4
Preface 5
Acknowledgements 6
Authors 7
Editors 8
Contributors 9
Paper 1 Questions 10
Paper 1 Answers 20
Paper 2 Questions 39
Paper 2 Answers 48
Paper 3 Questions 67
Paper 3 Answers 79
Paper 4 Questions 101
Paper 4 Answers 117
Thank you 132

Preface

Dermatology is a subject that is poorly taught in medical schools despite that skin conditions are the most common type of presentation seen in practice. This is reflected in students often scoring poorly in the dermatology section of their exams, and doctors are shy of making skin diagnoses.

The General Medical Council (GMC) is introducing a new Medical Licensing Assessment (MLA) for all medical students graduating from 2023 to meet a standard threshold for safe practice. They have released a content map which this book is tailored around.

This book is the first in providing a comprehensive summary of the new MLA curriculum through 180 multiple-choice questions (MCQ) with detailed explanations of the relevant conditions. Moreover, we have added high yield exam questions that are not included in the MLA curriculum but apply to medical school exams. This book also contains questions and notes on basic science, anatomy and physiology of the skin.

This book was co-authored by a medical student who is familiar with the level of detail required to excel in dermatology medical exams and a junior doctor who recently succeeded in his final medical school exams and has already co-authored a book called 'The Duke Elder Exam of Ophthalmology – the comprehensive guide for success'. Furthermore, the book was edited and reviewed by one consultant dermatologist, specialty register and a clinical fellow in dermatology. We firmly believe that this resource will help a student succeed in their dermatology exams.

Acknowledgements

We are grateful to the dermatology imaging team at Ninewells Hospital and in particular, Mr. Andrew Coon, for providing us with photographs of dermatological conditions to aid visual understanding of the diseases. We want to thank all the patients who have allowed us to utilize their photos in this book. We also want to express our gratitude to Dr Iman Kotb, Dr Amina Khalid and Dr Sanaa Butt who were extremely helpful and patient in the process of writing this book. Also, a big thank you to the latter Doctors for taking the time to review this book.

Authors

Abigail Johnston

Abigail just completed her third year in medical school at Dundee. She is currently undertaking a BMSc in Medical Education this year and her Associate Fellowship of the Higher Education Academy (AFHEA). Abigail has co-founded Bridging the Gap Academy, which is a medical, educational platform. She has a keen interest in breast surgery, being a regional lead for the National Surgery Teaching Society (NSTS). Currently, she is undertaking various projects, including looking at the newest technique in breast surgery reconstruction named lateral intercostal artery perforator flap (LICAP). Abigail is the student representative for the Association of Medical Education in Europe's (AMEE) 2021 Conference Advisory Group.

Dr Mostafa Khalil (MBChB)

Mostafa is a General Surgery Clinical Fellow at Ninewells Hospital and Medical school. He was awarded the prize for the highest mark in his Medical School Finals examination in 2018. He also ranked 5th in the UK in the national prize examination named the Duke Elder Exam of Ophthalmology. He later co-authored a book titled The Duke Elder Exam of Ophthalmology: A Comprehensive Guide for Success. Along with Abigail, he co-founded Bridging the Gap Academy.

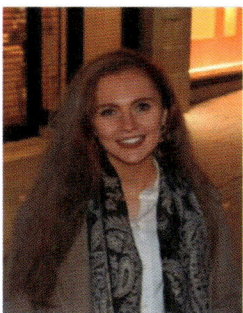
Abigail Johnston

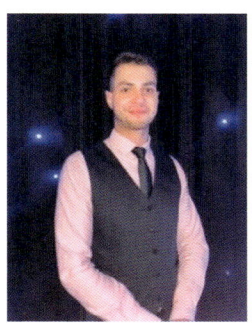
Mostafa Khalil

Editors

Dr Iman Kotb

Dr Kotb is a senior dermatology registrar in Aberdeen Royal Infirmary. She graduated from Mansoura Medical School and completed three years training program in dermatology concluded with a master's degree from Mansoura University in Egypt. At the University of Aberdeen, she achieved a PhD and finished the Royal College of Physicians exams, and the Dermatology Specialty exam before securing a National UK specialty training number. Dr Kotb was a co-investigator in clinical trials, and her research interest is in understanding the immune mechanisms underlying skin diseases. Also, she is an associate editor for the Skin Health and Disease journal.

Dr Amina Khalid

Dr Khalid is a consultant dermatologist at Ninewells Hospital and Medical School, Dundee. She has specialist interest in surgical Dermatology and cutaneous lymphoma. She has the following qualifications: MBBS, MRCP, MRCP Derm, Dip Dermatology Glasgow.

Dr Sanaa Butt

Dr Butt is a clinical fellow doctor in Dermatology department at Ninewells Hospital and Medical School, Dundee. She has a keen interest in medical education and dermatological skin surgery. She has the following qualifications: BMBS, MRCP.

Contributors

Cara Richardson

Alicia Binning

Claire Orr

Dr Esther McNeill

Paper 1 Questions

1. What part of the body does tinea unguium affect?

    A. Scalp
    B. Trunk, legs and arms
    C. Feet
    D. Nails

2. What organism is responsible for pityriasis versicolor?

    A. Trichophyton tonsurans
    B. Malassezia furfur
    C. Trichophyton rubrum
    D. Candida

3. A 17-year-old woman presents to the GP with extreme vulval itching and erythema. The patient also describes a 'cottage cheese', non-offensive discharge. She has no past medical history; except she is on the combined oral contraceptive pill.

What is the most likely diagnosis?

    A. Chlamydia
    B. Gonorrhoea
    C. Bacterial vaginosis
    D. Candidiasis

4. What human papillomavirus (HPV) is responsible for most foot warts?

    A. HPV 1
    B. HPV 2
    C. HPV 6 and 11
    D. HPV 16 and 18

5. A 22-year-old pregnant woman presents with dysuria and an irritating rash. She has a red, tender vesicular rash on her vulva. The GP does a urine dipstick test, which shows blood and white cells.
What is the most appropriate treatment?

A. Clotrimazole
B. Topical aciclovir
C. Oral aciclovir
D. Fluconazole

6. A mother of a three-year-old girl who is known to have eczema presents with worsening skin. Her mum says it has been occurring for about a week and that she is not her usual self. On examination, she has widespread clusters of itchy blisters and painful punched out erosions on her face, trunk and limbs. She also feels febrile.

What is the most likely diagnosis?

A. Erythema multiforme
B. Exacerbation of eczema
C. Eczema herpeticum
D. Herpes simplex encephalitis

7. A 4-year-old girl presents with erythematous, painful, and swollen gums. There are also vesicles in the gums. Following the examination, the patient has a fever, malaise and cervical lymphadenopathy.

What is the most likely diagnosis?

A. Primary gingivostomatitis
B. Herpes simplex virus -1
C. Eczema herpeticum
D. Dermatitis Herpetiformis

8. What is the causative organism of chickenpox?

A. Herpes simplex virus
B. Varicella zoster virus
C. Staphylococcus aureus
D. Coxsackievirus

9. What are "pearly-pink umbilicated papules" characteristic of?

   A. Herpangina
   B. Molluscum contagiosum
   C. Hand, foot and mouth disease (HFMD)
   D. Squamous cell carcinoma

10. What is the most common causative organism for hand, foot and mouth disease (HFMD)?

    A. Coxsackie A16 virus
    B. Parvovirus B19
    C. Herpes simplex
    D. Group A haemolytic streptococci

11. A patient presents with pityriasis Rosea. What most commonly occurs before this condition?

    A. Sunlight
    B. Bacterial infection
    C. Viral infection
    D. Antibiotics use

12. What is Bowen's disease?

    A. Type of basal cell carcinoma
    B. Type of actinic keratosis
    C. A precursor to squamous cell carcinoma
    D. A precursor to basal cell carcinoma

13. How often does invasive squamous cell carcinoma (SCC) arise in a patch of Bowen's or intraepidermal SCC?

    A. No, it never happens
    B. It is infrequent
    C. It is common
    D. It always happens

14. A 75-year-old Caucasian gentleman with type I skin attends his GP. He presents with many small, crusty white/yellow scaly lesions scattered on his scalp, with associated erythema. Following discussion, you find out that he used to be a 'sun-worshiper' and rarely wore sun cream.

What is the most likely diagnosis of this patient?

- A. Squamous cell carcinoma
- B. Basal cell carcinoma
- C. Actinic keratoses
- D. Keratoacanthoma (KA)

15. Is there a risk of transformation from actinic keratosis to squamous cell carcinoma?

- A. No, it never happens
- B. Small risk
- C. It is common
- D. It always happens

16. A 56-year-old man, with type I skin, presents with a 7-week history of a rapidly growing lesion on his left forearm. The appearance of the lesion has changed over two weeks from a small red papule to a bigger raised solid nodule filled with keratin.

What is the most likely diagnosis?

- A. Keratoacanthoma (KA)
- B. Seborrhoeic keratosis
- C. Pyoderma gangrenosum
- D. Malignant melanoma

17. Does basal cell carcinoma commonly metastasise?

- A. It always metastasises
- B. Yes, it commonly metastasises
- C. Sometimes it metastasises
- D. It very rarely metastasises

18. Name a precursor of squamous cell carcinoma

    A. Bowen's disease
    B. Keratoacanthoma
    C. Ephelides
    D. Actinic Lentigines

19. What is the most common skin cancer?

    A. Squamous cell carcinoma
    B. Malignant melanoma
    C. Keratoacanthoma
    D. Basal cell carcinoma

20. What type of melanoma predominantly has a rapid vertical growth phase?

    A. Superficial spreading melanoma
    B. Acral/mucosal lentiginous melanoma
    C. Lentigo maligna melanoma
    D. Nodular melanoma

21. Where is acral lentiginous melanoma most commonly found?

    A. Limbs and trunks
    B. On palms and soles of feet, or nails
    C. Sun-damaged skin of head and neck
    D. On any sun-exposed areas

22. A 85-year-old gentleman is diagnosed with mild actinic keratosis. What management is the most suitable for this patient?

    A. Ketoconazole
    B. Topical tacrolimus
    C. Benzoyl peroxide
    D. Topical 5-Fluorouracil

23. What is the most common subtype of melanoma?

    A. Superficial spreading melanoma
    B. Acral/mucosal lentiginous melanoma
    C. Lentigo maligna melanoma
    D. Nodular melanoma

24. A 35-year-old woman presents to the GP. On examination, you notice around 20 atypical naevi on her back. She says she has noticed no change in her moles. There has been no bleeding or itching. However, you accidentally spotted a mole with an irregular border, and it is 7 * 4 mm in size.

What is the most appropriate course of action?

    A. Review in three months
    B. Refer routinely to dermatology for photo mapping
    C. Refer urgently under the two-week rule to dermatology
    D. Advise sun protection & take a digital photo for her records

25. What is the most appropriate way to diagnose a suspected melanoma?

    A. Shave biopsy
    B. By appearance
    C. Full-thickness excisional biopsy
    D. Punch biopsy

26. Where is Breslow thickness (mm) measured from?

    A. The granular layer of epidermis down to the deepest point of invasion
    B. The basal layer of epidermis down to the deepest point of invasion
    C. Melanocytes down to the deepest point of invasion
    D. Keratin layer of epidermis down to the deepest point of invasion

27. Select the statement which is true of eczema.

    A. Eczema is contagious and spreads through physical contact

- B. Genetic background is a strong predictor of eczema
- C. Eczema often occurs as a lone condition
- D. Most people develop eczema during their adulthood

28. What is mycosis Fungoides?

   A. A cutaneous B-cell lymphoma
   B. A cutaneous T-cell lymphoma
   C. Psoriasis
   D. Tinea corporis

29. A 25-year-old man presents to his GP with erythematous, well-defined scaly plaques on the extensor surfaces of his elbows. On examination, you notice the scale on the plaques has a silvery colour and that there are little spots of bleeding on his forearm, where the scale has come off. You notice that his fingernails have no noticeable abnormalities. He says that he has been well and has had no recent infections.

What is the most likely diagnosis?

   A. Flexural psoriasis
   B. Plaque psoriasis
   C. Guttate psoriasis
   D. Pustular psoriasis

30. A patient presents with widespread painful erythema over 90% of his whole body. The skin is also warm to touch.

What subtype of psoriasis is this most likely to be?

   A. Erythrodermic psoriasis
   B. Palmoplantar pustulosis
   C. Pustular psoriasis
   D. Plaque psoriasis

31. What is characteristic of psoriasis on histopathology?

   A. Acanthosis
   B. Papillomatosis

C. Parakeratosis
   D. Spongiosis

32. The Koebner phenomenon occurs in psoriasis. What is the Koebner phenomenon?

   A. Psoriasis scales are scraped off, causing small bleeds
   B. Psoriasis scales in areas exposed to sunlight
   C. Psoriasis lesions where there has never been any trauma
   D. Psoriasis lesions appear at sites where there has been trauma

33. What is the first line for plaque psoriasis?

   A. Coal tar (once or twice daily) or a potential corticosteroid (twice daily).
   B. Vitamin D analogue twice daily.
   C. Potent corticosteroid (once daily) + Vitamin D analogue (once daily). One in the morning, the other in the evening, for four weeks. Or a combination of calcipotriol/betamethasone (in one product) OD for four weeks.
   D. Narrowband Ultraviolet Blight three times a week

34. A 46-year-old female presents with itchy, violaceous papules on the flexor aspects of her wrists and her lumbar region. Before this, she was well and had no other health conditions.

What other feature may you expect to find in this condition?

   A. Macroscopic haematuria
   B. Mucous membrane involvement
   C. Onycholysis
   D. Scaling of lesions

35. What are Wickham's striae?

   A. Pinkish lines visible on the papules of lichen planus.
   B. Purplish lines visible on the papules of lichen planus.
   C. Violet lines visible on the papules of lichen planus.
   D. Whitish lines visible on the papules of lichen planus.

36. What histopathology is characteristic of Lichen planus?

    A. Hyperkeratosis and parakeratosis
    B. Spongiosis
    C. Papillomatosis
    D. Irregular, saw-tooth acanthosis

37. What is the mainstay of treatment for localised lichen planus?

    A. Topical steroid cream
    B. Systemic steroids, e.g., prednisolone
    C. Narrow band UVB
    D. Topical immunomodulators e.g., imiquimod

38. A 23-year-old female presents to her GP with a butterfly rash that is on her cheeks and nose. Following further questioning, she complains that she has been losing some hair also.

What is the most likely diagnosis?

    A. Acne rosacea
    B. Erythema multiforme
    C. Alopecia areata
    D. Systemic lupus erythematosus (SLE)

39. Which of the following is not a cutaneous feature of systemic lupus erythematosus?

    A. Discoid lupus
    B. Alopecia
    C. Livedo reticularis
    D. Vitiligo

40. A 36-year-old man attends his GP. In just over two weeks, a painful, erythematous lesion on his skin, on the dorsal aspect of his hand has appeared. On examination, the lesion is circular. There is no relevant past medical history apart from using NSAIDs.

What is the most likely diagnosis?

A. Erythema multiforme (EM)
B. Toxic Epidermal necrolysis
C. Neurofibromatosis
D. Contact allergic dermatitis

41. Erythema multiforme is most commonly triggered by what infection?

A. Human papillomavirus
B. Herpes simplex virus
C. Coxsackievirus A16
D. Parvovirus B19

42. "A rare and acute skin condition where the skin becomes sheet-like, and there is associated mucosal loss. The skin condition takes up >30% of a patient's skin".

This statement best describes what condition?

A. Toxic epidermal necrolysis (TEN)
B. Steven-Johnson Syndrome
C. Hand, foot and mouth disease
D. Erythema infectiosum

43. A 24-year-old female presents to A&E with significant blistering and a necrotic skin rash that is widespread across her skin. On examination, this includes the mucous membranes too. The patient tells you that she was treated for an infection a week ago by her GP.

What medication is most likely to have triggered this rash?

A. Nitrofurantoin
B. Metronidazole
C. Aciclovir
D. Co-amoxiclav

44. A 26-year-old man presents to the GP with vitiligo. He has read that because of his condition; he is at risk of other autoimmune diseases.

What condition is he most at risk of?

- A. Type 2 diabetes
- B. Childhood asthma
- C. Addison's disease
- D. Toxic multi-nodular goitre

45. What description <u>best</u> describes vitiligo?

- A. Loss of melanocytes
- B. Loss of melanin
- C. Increase in melanocytes
- D. Increase in melanin

Paper 1 Answers

Question 1
Correct Answer: D

Tinea unguium is a fungal infection of the nails.

Tinea (a.k.a. ringworm of the skin) is a dermatophyte fungal infection (dermatophyte are fungi that need keratin for growth). The most common cause of tinea capitis is Trichophyton tonsurans. Diagnosis is usually clinical or skin scraping/nail clippings for microscopy. Treatment depends on the degree of infection. If small/localised infection: clotrimazole cream. For extensive/stubborn infection: oral terbinafine or oral itraconazole. Suppose nails are involved: Amorolfine (nail lacquer) or terbinafine (oral). The differential diagnosis of tinea unguium includes nail psoriasis, Candidiasis, subungual wart and lichen planus.

Classification of Tinea:

Type of Tinea	Parts of the body affected

Tinea capitis	Scalp
Tinea corporis	Trunk, legs and arm
Tinea pedis (more common in adolescent males)	Feet
Tinea unguium	Nails
Tinea barbae	Beard
Tinea manuum	Hands
Tinea cruris	Groin

Question 2
Correct Answer: B

Pityriasis Versicolor is a superficial fungal infection of the skin due to *Malassezia furfur*. More common in humid conditions and males. Often it presents on the trunks of the patients. In Caucasian skin, it shows as brown/pink round scaly patches. For racially pigmented skin, there is hypopigmentation. An essential difference between Vitiligo and Pityriasis Versicolor is that Pityriasis Versicolor has a fine-scale visible with the naked eye and wood's light gives a yellow fluorescence (can be negative for P. Versicolor if scales are removed, e.g., shower the day before). Management is a topical antifungal: ketoconazole shampoo. If no response to treatment, send scrapings for microscopy and treat with oral itraconazole.

Question 3
Correct Answer: D

This patient has Candidiasis. It is the most common yeast infection affecting the skin. *Candida* is part of the normal vaginal flora, but sometimes it colonises an area resulting in a severe itch. It is more common in immunocompromised individuals (HIV, diabetics), broad-spectrum use antibiotics, pregnancy and the use of COCP. Diagnosis is usually clinical. Treatment includes clotrimazole cream/pessary or oral fluconazole. Chlamydia is an STI that often is asymptomatic or presents with dysuria and vaginal/urethral discharge. Gonorrhoea presents with yellow/green discharge and dysuria. Bacterial vaginosis is an overgrowth of organisms such as *Gardnerella vaginalis* and it presents as a vaginal discharge that is 'fishy' and offensive, with characteristic clue cells.

Question 4
Correct Answer: A

HPV 1 is responsible for foot warts.

HPV type	Associated lesion
1	Foot warts
2	Hand warts
6 and 11	Genital warts
16 and 18	Cervical cancer

Common warts usually are dome-shaped nodules or papules with papilliferous surfaces. In exams often described as "cauliflower appearance". Verrucas are essentially warts on the plantar aspects of the feet. A patient's body weight causes them to grow into the dermis. Management: 1st line Salicylic acid. 2nd line: Cryotherapy (freezing) or Imiquimod. Also, laser, electrosurgery with local anaesthesia. It is important to note that HPV in renal transplant patients has been linked to skin cancer, especially squamous cell carcinoma. HPV 16 and 18 are significant risk factors for cervical cancer.

Question 5
Correct Answer: C

This patient has genital herpes simplex virus (HSV). During any stage of pregnancy, it is recommended that oral (or intravenous) aciclovir is used. Topical aciclovir is used more for localised HSV infection. However, if HSV infection is more widespread/systemic, then oral aciclovir is used. Clotrimazole is an antifungal used to treat conditions like Candidiasis, therefore would be ineffective in HSV as it has a viral cause. The same applies to fluconazole which is also an antifungal infection.

Herpes simplex is a common blistering viral infection of the skin. There are two strains of HSV. HSV-1 and HSV-2. HSV-1 is primarily facial, and non-genital (normally childhood-onset) and HSV-2 is mainly genital (adult-onset). However, there is some cross over. Following primary infection of HSV, the virus remains dormant within the dorsal root ganglion. Reactivation can occur due to sunlight, stress or immunosuppression.

Question 6
Correct Answer: C

Eczema herpeticum is a disseminated viral infection of the skin caused by HSV-1 or HSV-2. It is more commonly seen in children with atopic eczema (it can also occur in other skin diseases, e.g. pemphigus vulgaris, darier disease, mycosis fungoides. Eczema herpeticum presents with a rapidly progressive painful rash, and on examination, there are monomorphic punched out erosions. This condition is a dermatological emergency, and therefore children should be considered for admission to receive IV aciclovir. Secondary bacterial infection with staphylococci or streptococci can occur and lead to impetigo and cellulitis. Confirmation of the diagnosis is by the viral swab. The bacterial swab should also be taken for culture and sensitivity as secondary bacterial infection is common. Erythema multiforme is a hypersensitivity reaction that is primarily triggered by infections and characterised by target lesions.

There is no mention of target lesions in the question making this improbable. An exacerbation of eczema is unlikely due to the patient not having a temperature. Herpes simplex encephalitis is a hot exam topic! The virus affects typically the temporal lobes giving focal features such as aphasia and also general features such as fever, headache, seizures and vomiting. The treatment is IV aciclovir. This patient has none of these symptoms.

Question 7
Correct Answer: A

The correct answer is primary gingivostomatitis. In this condition, the vesicles will rupture into painful, large, ulcerated areas. It commonly affects children aged six months to 6 years. These lesions will spontaneously heal in 1 to 2 weeks. Treatment is supportive. HSV-1 causes cold sores, and usually, the child isn't systemically unwell. Eczema herpeticum presents typically in children who have pre-existing eczema and develop herpes simplex virus. Dermatitis Herpetiformis is an autoimmune blistering skin condition associated with coeliac disease. The skin lesions are on the extensor aspects of the body and are itchy; these features are missing in this four-year-old.

Question 8
Correct Answer: B

The varicella zoster virus causes chickenpox. The primary infection is called varicella (chickenpox). If the dormant virus in the dorsal root ganglia is reactivated, this will cause zoster (shingles). 90% of patients are affected before adolescence. With chickenpox, the first feature is often pyrexia. The vesicles appear over 3-5 days polymorphic- mainly on the neck, head and trunk. The lesions are very itchy, following a course of papule, vesicle, pustule and crust. Most cases of chickenpox are self-limiting. If a patient is immunocompromised or pregnant, anti-viral treatment should be given as soon as possible. Shingles is an acutely painful dermatomal skin rash caused by reactivation of VZV.

Shingles are more common in the elderly and cause a rash for 2-3 days, followed by pain in a dermatomal nature. A vaccine is offered to all patients aged 70-79 years; it is live-attenuated. First-line management is oral aciclovir.

Herpes simplex viruses cause cold sores and genital herpes. Staph aureus is a causative organism for cellulitis and impetigo. Herpangina is a painful mouth infection caused by coxsackieviruses, typically coxsackievirus A. It usually occurs in children in the summer.

Question 9
Correct Answer: B
Pearly-pink umbilicated papules are characteristic of Molluscum contagiosum. This is an infection caused by a poxvirus and appears as clusters of small rounded umbilicated papules, 1-6 mm in size and commonly affects children and young adults under the age of 10. Lesions can be seen anywhere on the body except the palms and soles. Molluscum contagiosum is self-limiting and will clear within 12-18 months. Herpangina is a painful mouth infection caused by coxsackieviruses, mainly coxsackievirus A. There are often red spots on the uvula, soft palate and tonsils, these then develop into a tiny grey-white papulovesicular rash. Usually resolves within 5-10 days.
Hand, foot and mouth disease is a viral infection that affects the mouth, hands and feet, characterised by blisters/ulcers. Squamous cell carcinoma (SCC) appears as a firm pink lump with a keratinised surface (not necessarily as sometimes it appears fleshy or exophytic mass or ulcer). SCC can be differentiated because it is more common in old age and immunosuppressed, painful, sun-exposed sites.

Question 10
Correct Answer: A

Coxsackie A16 virus is the most common causative organism for HFMD. Other common causes include coxsackie A10 virus and enterovirus 71. Parvovirus B19 is responsible for erythema infectiosum, also known as 'slapped cheek syndrome' or fifths disease. It presents as a 'slapped cheek' rash spreading to the proximal arms and the extensor surfaces. They are associated with fever and lethargy. Herpes simplex causes cold sores and genital herpes. Group A haemolytic streptococci is a reaction to the erythrogenic toxins that cause scarlet fever. Scarlet fever presents as fever, tonsillitis, 'strawberry tongue' and a rash (fine punctate erythema sparing the area around the mouth (circumoral pallor)).

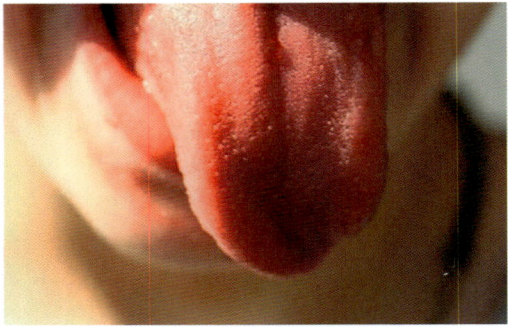

Figure 1: Strawberry tongue

Question 11
Correct Answer: C

A viral infection usually precedes Pityriasis Rosea. Sunlight can trigger infections such as Acne Rosacea and cold sores caused by HSV-1. Streptococcal throat infections can trigger guttate psoriasis. Antibiotics are not the correct answer as they are not a known trigger of Pityriasis Rosea. Pityriasis Rosea is an acute rash, and its aetiology is not fully understood. However, it is thought that HHV-7 may have a role.
The characteristic buzzword is herald patch (generally on the trunk). Erythematous, oval, scaly patches follow the herald patch creating a 'fir-tree' rash. It is self-limiting and lasts typically 12 weeks.

Question 12
Correct Answer: C

Bowen's disease is a precursor to squamous cell carcinoma. Common exam questions will be present with a woman over 60 years old, with small patches of red scaly skin, in areas of sun-exposed skin (often lower legs in elderly women). Risk factors for Bowen's disease include long term sun-exposure, sunbeds, immunosuppression, type I and II skin types and human papillomavirus infection. Bowen's disease is derived from keratinocytes of the epidermis. Management includes surgical excision, imiquimod cream, 5% 5-Fluorouracil cream, liquid nitrogen cryotherapy and photodynamic therapy. Other names for Bowen's disease are SCC in situ or intraepidermal SCC

Question 13
Correct Answer: B

The transformation of Bowen's disease into squamous cell carcinoma is infrequent (5%).

Question 14
Correct Answer: C

This patient has actinic keratosis (AK), also known as solar keratosis. It is rare for a single AK lesion to change into SCC, but patients with more than 10 AK lesions are at increased risk to develop SCC. Actinic keratosis is very common in elderly Caucasians and presents as single or multiple patches that are usually rough, scaly and hyperkeratotic areas. The most standard sites are sun-exposed areas. Risk factors comprise of sun damage, type I and II skin types and immunosuppression. Actinic keratosis results from abnormal keratinocyte growth due to DNA damage. Management includes imiquimod cream, 5% 5-Fluorouracil cream, liquid nitrogen, cryotherapy and photodynamic therapy.

Squamous cell carcinoma presents as a hyperkeratotic lesion with crusting and ulceration. Basal cell carcinoma is a translucent or pearly rodent ulcer with telangiectasia and rolled raised edges. Keratoacanthoma (KA) is a rapidly growing lesion, followed by spontaneous resolution over 4-6 months.

Question 15
Correct Answer: B

There is a small risk of transformation of actinic keratosis (AK) to squamous cell carcinoma (SCC). It is rare for a single AK lesion to change into SCC, but patients with more than 10 AK lesions are at increased risk to develop SCC (10 to 15%).

Question 16
Correct Answer: A

Keratoacanthoma (KA) is usually a solitary round, firm reddish or skin-coloured papule/nodule that rapidly changes into a dome-shaped nodule with a smooth, shiny surface. A central crater of ulceration may develop, or a keratin plug like a horn. It often mimics squamous cell carcinoma. KA grows more rapidly than squamous cell carcinoma (SCC). It is more common in the elderly, Caucasian males with a history of increased sun exposure. Diagnosis requires an excisional biopsy to rule out SCC. Gold standard treatment is complete excision. Seborrhoeic keratosis has a stuck-on appearance and is benign epidermal skin lesions seen in older people. Pyoderma gangrenosum is a painful ulcerative skin condition usually associated with systemic diseases. Malignant melanoma is a brown or black skin lesion with an irregular border, 2 or 3 mixed colours, and and abnormal pigment network on dermoscopy.

Question 17
Correct Answer: D

Basal cell cancer very rarely metastases. Basal cell carcinomas are common, locally malignant basal cell tumours. They are slow-growing. Risk factors include Caucasian, elderly (however the incidence is increasing in younger populations), sun damage, immunosuppression, Gorlin syndrome, Albinism and Xeroderma pigmentosum. Classical presentation: translucent or pearly rodent ulcers with telangiectasia and rolled raised edges. There are different sub-types: Nodular (most common and a.k.a. "rodent ulcer"), superficial, morphoeic (can infiltrate) and pigmented. Diagnosis is via a biopsy - excisional biopsy (with 4 mm margin) for nodular types or a small diagnostic punch biopsy for the superficial type. Management is usually surgical excision. Superficial BCC is generally treated with Imiquimod cream, liquid nitrogen cryotherapy, photodynamic therapy or 5-fluorouracil cream.

Question 18
Correct Answer: A

Bowen's disease and actinic keratosis can be a precursor to squamous cell carcinoma. Squamous cell carcinoma is a non-melanoma skin cancer that arises from the keratinising cells of the epidermis. Squamous cell carcinoma can spread to local lymph nodes. It usually presents as a hyperkeratotic lesion with crusting and ulceration. Diagnosis is via an excisional biopsy (with 4-6 margin). The gold standard is surgical excision with 5 mm margin and confirmation of clearance by histology. Keratoacanthoma is regarded as a variant of the keratinocyte or squamous cell carcinoma. Ephelides are freckles. Actinic Lentigines are also known as "age spots or solar keratosis". These are flat patches of pigmented skin.

Question 19
Correct Answer: D

The most common type of skin cancer is basal cell carcinoma. The second most common is squamous cell carcinoma. Although melanoma has had a 134% increase since the 1990s, it is not the most common type of skin cancer.

Question 20

Correct Answer: D

A rapid vertical growth phase characterises nodular melanoma. Lesions with radial growth phase (with epidermis) +/- vertical growth phase (dermal invasion) includes superficial spreading melanoma, acral/mucosal lentiginous melanoma and lentigo maligna melanoma. Melanoma is a malignant tumour of melanocytes. Risk factors of melanoma include previous melanoma, family history, type I and II skin types, sun damage, albinism, xeroderma pigmentosum, immunosuppression and multiple atypical or dysplastic naevi.

Question 21
Correct Answer: B

Acral lentiginous melanoma is found on the palm and soles of feet, or nails. Notably, it is rare in Caucasians, and it arises from pigmented lesions. Nodular melanoma is found most commonly on trunks and limbs. They are characterised by rapid vertical growth phase, and this is why it is the most aggressive type of melanoma. Lentigo maligna melanoma is a malignant melanoma that develops in a long-standing lentigo maligna. They are often found on the head and neck of an elderly person who has spent many years in an outdoor occupation or sunbeds. Superficial spreading melanoma is flat irregular pigmented skin lesions that appear most commonly on the limbs and trunk.

Question 22
Correct Answer: D

Topical diclofenac is used in the management of mild actinic keratosis. Benzoyl peroxide is part of the acne treatment. Ketoconazole is used in the treatment of fungal infections. Topical tacrolimus can be utilised in the treatment of eczema.

Question 23
Correct Answer: A

The most common subtype of melanoma is superficial spreading melanoma.

Question 24
Correct Answer: C

This woman most likely has melanoma, and therefore they should be referred urgently under the two-week rule to dermatology. The criteria for a referral here are an irregular shape (major) and a diameter of 7 mm (minor). In the question, the woman says she has not noticed a difference; however, the moles are on her back, and therefore she is unlikely to see their change in appearance. Not referring the patient immediately to dermatology would be inappropriate because melanoma has an ability to metastasis via the lymphatic system to local lymph nodes, or via the bloodstream to other organs. Common sites for metastases include lymph nodes, lung, liver, brain and bone.

Question 25
Correct Answer: C

A full-thickness excisional biopsy is required for the diagnosis of a suspected melanoma, with an initial 2mm margin of normal skin around the melanoma. If melanoma is confirmed, then all patients are offered a wider excision. They may be considered for a sentinel lymph node biopsy dependent on the Breslow thickness and the multi-disciplinary team discussion.

Question 26
Correct Answer: A

Breslow thickness is a measure from the granular layer of the epidermis down to the deepest point of invasion. The Breslow thickness determines the prognosis of melanoma.

Question 27
Correct Answer: B

A patient's genetic background is a strong predictor of eczema (family history of atopy in general, not just skin). Eczema is not contagious and frequently presents with other conditions. Up to 80% of children with atopic dermatitis go on to develop hay fever or asthma. Eczema is more common in children, and most individuals develop this condition within the first five years of their life.

Question 28
Correct Answer: B

Mycosis Fungoides is a type of cutaneous T-cell lymphoma (CTCL), and it is the most common type of CTCL. Often it is diagnosed at 55-60 years old, and it is most prominently distributed asymmetrically in the "bathing suit" area, although it can affect any part of the skin. There are 3 phases: patch phase, plaque phase and mycotic/tumour phase. For a definite diagnosis of mycosis fungoides, a skin biopsy is needed, which shows Pautrier's microabscesses and a band-like upper dermal infiltrate. Sézary cells on blood film (atypical lymphocytes), a CT/MRI may be used to see if other parts of the body are affected. It is rarely curable; however, the progression of the disease is usually slow.

Question 29
Correct Answer: B

This patient has plaque psoriasis; this is the most common subtype of psoriasis. Plaque psoriasis is a well-demarcated pink or red, flaky plaque, +/- silvery-white scaly layer on the top that makes it feel rough. Most commonly occur on the knees, elbows and the lower back (extensor distribution). It can also appear on the scalp and nails. Flexural psoriasis is found on the flexor surface of the body, rather than the extensor surface in plaque psoriasis. Guttate psoriasis is another type of psoriasis, and it usually occurs 7-10 days post-viral URTI infection or post-streptococcal infection. It is more commonly found in children and young adults.

There is characteristic "teardrop-shaped", scaly plaques located on the limbs and trunk. Pustular psoriasis presents as widespread erythematous skin with multiple pustules, and the skin is tender. Pustular psoriasis is a rare form and is most commonly found on the flexures and genitalia.

Question 30
Correct Answer: A

Erythrodermic psoriasis presents as widespread painful erythema over 90% of the total body area. The skin is also warm to touch. This condition is one of the dermatological emergencies, and therefore, hospital admission is necessary because it can affect the patient's ability to control their body temperature and dehydration. Palmoplantar pustulosis affects the soles of the feet and the palms of the hands. It presents as sterile pustules, (does not contain bacteria and it is not infectious). Usually, the skin around the pustules is red and tender. Pustular psoriasis presents as pustules on a background of red and tender skin. Plaque psoriasis presents as plaques mainly on the extensor surfaces. Flexural psoriasis is glazed non-scaly plaques (due to friction), and it affects the submammary areas, groin, axillae and natal cleft.

Question 31
Correct Answer: C

Parakeratosis is characteristic of psoriasis; this is the retention of nuclei in the keratin layer and is a sign that the epithelium is turning over too quickly. Spongiosis is oedema fluid in the epidermis; this is characteristic of eczema. Acanthosis is the increased thickness of the epithelium. Papillomatosis is irregular epithelial thickness. Hyperkeratosis is the increased thickness of the epithelium, and it is also present in psoriasis.

Question 32
Correct Answer: D

Koebner phenomenon is where psoriasis lesions appear at sites where there has initially been skin trauma. This is a feature of psoriasis. Answer A describes Auspitz's sign which also occurs in psoriasis. Psoriasis lesions may improve by exposure to sunlight.

Question 33
Correct Answer: C

The first-line treatment for psoriasis is a potent corticosteroid (once daily) and Vitamin D analogue (once daily). One in the morning, the other in the evening, for four weeks. All patients are given emollients as well- if the skin has a thick scale, emollient helps to descale and optimise penetration of topical treatments. 2nd line treatment is answer B. So, if after eight weeks and no improvement, give vitamin D analogue twice daily. 3rd line treatment is answer A. So, after eight to twelve weeks, if no improvement then offers either: coal tar (once or twice daily) or a potential corticosteroid (twice daily).

Secondary care management:
Reasons for referral to secondary care include a progression of psoriasis, no response to treatment after compliance with topical treatment for six months, or side effects of topical therapy.
Phototherapy: Narrowband, Ultraviolet B light, is the treatment of choice three times a week (answer D).

Systemic therapies, e.g., methotrexate (usually if joints are involved). It is important to remember that methotrexate is contraindicated in pregnancy and requires careful monitoring of liver function tests (LFTs) due to its hepatotoxicity and full blood count (FBC) for myelosuppression.

Question 34
Correct Answer: B

The answer is mucous membrane involvement – these are commonly affected in lichen planus. This patient has Lichen Planus, which is an autoimmune disease. It is known as the **P** disease: **p**lanus, **p**urple, **p**ruritic, **p**apular, **p**olygonal rash on flexor surfaces. Lichen planus is commonly found on the flexor surfaces of the upper extremities, mucous membranes and genitalia. It is characterised by purple/violet, flat and shiny papules. Typically lichen planus is diagnosed clinically; however, a skin biopsy may be taken to confirm.

Question 35
Correct Answer: D

Wickham's striae are whitish lines visible on the papules of lichen planus. As well as these striae present in lichen planus, there are also nail involvement - ridging, dystrophy, pitting and hyperkeratosis.

Question 36
Correct Answer: D

Irregular saw-tooth acanthosis is characteristic of Lichen planus. There are also bank-like lymphocytic infiltrate at the **DEJ**. Acanthosis is the increased thickness of the epithelium. Hyperkeratosis and parakeratosis are both found in psoriasis. Hyperkeratosis is increased thickness of the epithelium, and parakeratosis is the persistence of nuclei in the keratin layer. Spongiosis is oedema fluid in the epidermis; this is characteristic of eczema. Papillomatosis is irregular epithelial thickness.

Question 37
Correct Answer: A

The mainstay of treatment for lichen planus is topical steroid cream. However, treatment is not always needed. Second-line treatment is answer B, systemic steroids, e.g., prednisolone. If there is little improvement after a course of steroids, then narrow band UVB may be considered (answer C). It is important to note that lesions may resolve spontaneously over 6-12 months. However, oral lesions may never completely resolve.

Question 38
Correct Answer: D

This patient with SLE has the characteristic butterfly rash on her cheeks and nose. Also, the patient is describing alopecia which is also present in SLE. SLE is a systemic autoimmune condition that affects the skin, joints, kidneys, lungs, heart and causes tiredness. It is 6x more common in women than men, and it usually develops in women aged 20-49. Acne rosacea is a chronic skin condition that affects the nose, cheeks but also the forehead. However, it presents as persistent erythema with pustules and papules. Erythema multiforme is a hypersensitivity reaction that is usually triggered by infections. Target lesions are characteristic of this condition. Alopecia areata is something to consider because the patient describes hair loss, however the butterfly rash points you towards SLE.

Question 39
Correct Answer: D

Vitiligo is not a characteristic cutaneous feature of SLE. Vitiligo is associated with autoimmune diseases such as type 1 diabetes mellitus, autoimmune thyroid disorders and Addison's disease. Photosensitivity alopecia, discoid lupus and livedo reticularis are cutaneous features of SLE. Discoid lupus is the most common form of cutaneous lupus.

Discoid presents as scaly, coin-like plaques on the face, scalp and ears. Livedo-reticularis is reticular reddish-blue discolouration of the skin, and it blanches on pressure.

Question 40
Correct Answer: A

Erythema multiforme presents as "target lesions", and these lesions show the Koebner phenomenon. The eruption usually starts in the extremities and may spread to the trunk. The lesions are initially well-circumscribed, erythematous round macules. EM is self-limiting and usually resolves over several weeks. EM is a hypersensitivity reaction that is triggered by infection (in 90% of cases) or drug (e.g. NSAIDs, penicillins, barbiturates and anticonvulsants). Its peak incidence is between 20-40 years old. Stevens-Johnson syndrome (SJS) and toxic epidermal necrolysis (TEN) - are a spectrum of diseases caused by medications. In toxic epidermal necrolysis (TEM) there is widespread full-thickness epidermal necrolysis that develops, with erythema and sloughing of the mucosa and skin. Neurofibromatosis has cafe au lait spots; however, these are a light-brown colour and ordinarily present on the trunk. Contact allergic dermatitis is a type IV hypersensitivity reaction that occurs in response to being exposed to a particular substance e.g., latex gloves, nickel or fragrances. There is no mention of any obvious specific allergen in the question making answer D unlikely.

Question 41
Correct Answer: B

Erythema is triggered by infections 90% of the time, most commonly by HSV. Human papillomavirus causes warts, verrucas, genital warts and cancers. Coxsackievirus A16 causes hand, foot and mouth disease. Parvovirus B19 is responsible for slapped cheek disease.

Question 42
Correct Answer: A

Toxic epidermal necrolysis is a life-threatening hypersensitivity reaction that affects the mucous and cutaneous membranes. Steven-Johnson Syndrome (SJS) affects individuals aged 10-30 y/o and has a higher incidence in patients with HIV. TEN and SJS are variants of the same condition. SJS affects <10% of the total body surface and TEN affects > 30% of the total body surface. For both these conditions, remove the causative drug and give supportive treatment. Hand, foot and mouth disease and erythema infectiosum are both childhood infections and are not associated with such a large proportion of the skin being affected.

Question 43
Correct Answer: D

This patient has toxic epidermal necrolysis. Several drugs are possible triggers of this condition. Of the possible medications above, co-amoxiclav is most likely to cause TEN than other treatments. Other drugs known to induce TEN include sulphonamides, phenytoin, allopurinol, carbamazepine, NSAIDs and penicillins (e.g., co-amoxiclav).

Question 44
Correct Answer: C

Vitiligo is associated with autoimmune conditions including Addison's disease, type 1 diabetes, pernicious anaemia, alopecia areata and autoimmune thyroid disorders.

Question 45
Correct Answer: A

Vitiligo is an autoimmune disease that causes white patches on the body due to the absence of melanocytes in the area of skin affected and therefore no melanin. It is not more common in one racial or ethnic group; it is simply more noticeable in darker skin tones. Vitiligo can affect anywhere on the body, but most commonly the face, neck, wrists and scalp are affected. It presents as well-demarcated, hypopigmented/white patches on the skin, often symmetrical. There is no associated itch or pain in this condition.

Paper 2 Questions

1. Which of the following is not an accepted treatment for preventing the spread/enlargement of white patches in vitiligo?

    A. Topical ketoconazole
    B. Topical corticosteroid
    C. Tacrolimus
    D. Pimecrolimus

2. A 39-year-old male presents with two small, well-demarcated areas of hair loss, on scalp examination, there were short, broken "exclamation mark" hairs. He says there are no other areas of loss of hair on his body.

What is the most likely diagnosis?

    A. Patchy alopecia
    B. Extensive alopecia
    C. Alopecia totalis
    D. Alopecia universalis

3. Porphyrias are a group of metabolic conditions where there is a problem in the production of what component?

    A. Iron
    B. Haem
    C. Porphyrin

D. Oxygen

4. What is the inheritance mode of most types of porphyrias?

    A. Autosomal dominant
    B. Autosomal recessive
    C. X-linked recessive
    D. Mitochondrial

5. What enzyme is deficient in acute intermittent porphyria?

    A. Uroporphyrinogen decarboxylase (UROD)
    B. Uroporphyrinogen III
    C. Porphobilinogen deaminase (PBGD)
    D. Protoporphyrin

6. In what condition is there a build-up of excess protoporphyrin?

    A. Acute intermittent porphyria
    B. Porphyria cutanea tarda
    C. Erythropoietic protoporphyria
    D. All types of porphyria

7. A 9-year-old child presents to the GP with her mother. The child is experiencing burning, redness and itching on the skin on exposure to the sun. There is no blistering or scarring.

Which porphyria most likely presents in this way?

    A. Acute intermittent porphyria
    B. Porphyria cutanea tarda
    C. Erythropoietic protoporphyria
    D. All types of porphyria

8. In what porphyria is there usually no family history?

    A. Acute intermittent porphyria
    B. Porphyria cutanea tarda

C. Erythropoietic protoporphyria
D. All types of porphyria

9. In which porphyria is there an autosomal dominant genetic mutation in the HMBS gene?

   A. Acute intermittent porphyria
   B. Porphyria cutanea tarda
   C. Erythropoietic protoporphyria
   D. All types of porphyria

10. What condition is due to a mutation on chromosome 16?

    A. Neurofibromatosis type 1
    B. Tuberous sclerosis
    C. Gorlin's syndrome
    D. Wilson's disease

11. What inheritance is Tuberous sclerosis typically?

    A. Autosomal dominant
    B. Autosomal recessive
    C. X-linked recessive
    D. Mitochondrial

12. Café-au-lait and axillary/inguinal freckling are characteristic of what condition?

    A. Tuberous sclerosis
    B. Gorlin's syndrome
    C. Xeroderma Pigmentosum (XP)
    D. Neurofibromatosis type 1

13. Subungual fibromas are most commonly associated with what condition?

    A. Tuberous sclerosis
    B. Neurofibromatosis type 2

C. Psoriasis
D. Rheumatoid arthritis

14. This condition presents typically in childhood. It is characterised by extreme photosensitivity, and they experience a high incidence of skin cancer at a very young age. The child will have marked freckling in sun-exposed areas before two years old and xerosis. There may be eye features.

This description most likely portrays what condition?

    A. Gorlin's syndrome
    B. Xeroderma pigmentosum
    C. Epidermolysis bullosa
    D. Albinism

15. What condition has a mutation in the nucleotide excision repair (NER) genes?

    A. Gorlin's syndrome
    B. Xeroderma pigmentosum
    C. Epidermolysis bullosa
    D. Albinism

16. What is the embryological origin of melanocytes?

    A. Ectoderm
    B. Mesoderm
    C. Neural crest
    D. Dermis

17. What are the Blaschko lines?

    A. Lines of normal skin development
    B. Lines of a normal pattern of nerves
    C. Lines of a normal pattern of blood vessels
    D. Lines of an abnormal pattern of blood vessels

18. What layer of the epidermis are Odland bodies (lamellar bodies) found in?

A. Stratum corneum
B. Stratum granulosum
C. Stratum spinosum
D. Stratum basale

19. Select the correct statement.

　　A. Pheomelanin is the darker pigment found in red hair
　　B. Pheomelanin is the lighter pigment found in black and brunette hair
　　C. Eumelanin is the lighter pigment found in black and brunette hair
　　D. Eumelanin is the darker pigment found in black and brunette hair

20. "Partial loss of pigment production". This statement best matches what condition?

　　A. Albinism
　　B. Vitiligo
　　C. Malignant melanoma
　　D. Nelson's syndrome

21. What are Merkel cells?

　　A. Thermoreceptors
　　B. Mechanoreceptors
　　C. Pain receptors
　　D. Photoreceptors

22. Where are Langerhans cells found?

　　A. Stratum corneum
　　B. Stratum granulosum
　　C. Stratum spinosum
　　D. Stratum basale

23. What sweat glands are found specifically in the axillae, pubic area, anus and nipple area?

1. Sebaceous gland
2. Apocrine gland
3. Eccrine gland
4. All glands

24. What does the pilosebaceous unit consist of?

    A. Hair, hair follicle, sebaceous gland and arrector pili muscle
    B. Hair, hair follicle, apocrine gland and arrector pili muscle
    C. Hair, hair follicle, eccrine gland and arrector pili muscle
    D. Hair, hair follicle and arrector pili muscle

25. Choose the correct statement for describing the stages of hair growth.

    A. Anagen is a growing phase; catagen is the resting phase
    B. Catagen is a resting phase; telogen is the involuting phase
    C. Anagen is a growing phase; catagen is the involuting phase
    D. Telogen is a growing phase; catagen is the resting phase

26. What condition is characterised by hair thinning in the telogen phase?

    A. Alopecia Areata
    B. Telogen Effluvium
    C. Androgenic Alopecia
    D. Virilisation

27. What do Meissner's corpuscles detect?

    A. Vibration and fine touch
    B. Heat
    C. Pain
    D. Pressure

28. What feature of skin is responsible for vitamin D metabolism?

    A. Fibroblasts
    B. Melanocytes

C. Basal cells
D. Keratinocytes

29. A patient usually burns, sometimes tans, what number on the Fitzpatrick scale best describes this?

   A. Number I on the Fitzpatrick scale
   B. Number II on the Fitzpatrick scale
   C. Number III on the Fitzpatrick scale
   D. Number V on the Fitzpatrick scale

30. Urticaria, angioedema, atopy (e.g., asthma, eczema and rhinitis) best match what statement?

   A. Immediate Hypersensitivity (IgE mediated)
   B. Antibody-dependent - IgG, IgM
   C. Immune Complex Reaction
   D. Delayed - Cell-mediated Th1 cells

31. Which of the following facts are true?

   A. The growth rate of toenails is quicker than fingernails.
   B. Toe and fingernails grow quicker in the winter than the summer.
   C. The hyponychium is the underlying free edge of the nail plate.
   D. The cuticle of the nail is an extension of the skin plate covering the nail bed.

32. What T helper cells are associated with psoriasis? Pick two answers.

   A. TH1
   B. TH2
   C. TH17
   D. TH10

33. "Protection against viruses and cancer". What immunological cell best suits this description?

   A. TH2 cells

B. TH1 cells
C. CD8+ (cytotoxic T) cells
D. B cells

34. On what cells are MHC class 2 most commonly found?

    A. CD8+ cells
    B. Macrophages and B cells
    C. B cells and CD8+ cells
    D. Macrophages and CD8 + cells

35. "Enables the organism to avoid host defence mechanisms". What type of bacterial virulence factor does this best match?

    A. Adhesion
    B. Modulin
    C. Aggressin
    D. Impedin

36. What type of skin therapeutic best describes "semisolid emulsion of oil in water; it contains an emulsifier and preservative"?

    A. Creams
    B. Ointments
    C. Lotion
    D. Gels

37. What type of skin therapeutic would be more suitable for very dry or hyperkeratotic areas?

    A. Creams
    B. Ointments
    C. Paste
    D. Foams

38. A "stuck on appearance" best describes what lesion?

    A. Basal cell papilloma
    B. Basal cell carcinoma
    C. Squamous cell carcinoma

D. Acne vulgaris

39. A 15-year-old boy had his first HPV vaccine today. Shortly after this, he develops facial swelling and a red, itchy rash. He is rushed to the hospital with paramedics and develops a bilateral expiratory wheeze, and his blood pressure is 75/52 mmHg. Using Gell and Coombs classification of hypersensitivity reactions, what type is this?

   A. Type I reaction
   B. Type II reaction
   C. Type III reaction
   D. Type IV reaction

40. A 54-year-old woman presents with a red, weeping rash on her wrist after she has bought a new watch. Using Gell and Coombs classification of hypersensitivity reactions, what type is this?

   A. Type I reaction
   B. Type II reaction
   C. Type III reaction
   D. Type IV reaction

41. Diagnosis of type IV hypersensitivity reactions is via what?

   A. Skin prick testing/challenge testing
   B. Patch testing
   C. Specific IgE testing (RAST)
   D. Serum mast cell tryptase

42. A 22-year-old male presents to his GP, having noticed that for the past week, he has had an itchy rash on both his elbows. On examination, many polygonal, flat papular lesions are 4mm in diameter on her elbows in the flexor surface; this is bilateral. What is the most likely diagnosis?

   A. Eczema
   B. Lichen planus
   C. Psoriasis
   D. Pityriasis alba

43. What is the infective agent relevant in acne?

    A. *Staphylococcus aureus*
    B. *Streptococcus pyogenes*
    C. *Staphylococcus epidermidis*
    D. *Propionibacterium acnes*

44. What condition is most commonly associated with acanthosis nigricans?

    A. Squamous cell carcinoma
    B. Basal cell carcinoma
    C. Rubella
    D. Gastric adenocarcinoma and type 2 diabetes

45. What is the Leser-Trélat sign?

    A. Metastasis of gastric carcinoma to unilateral ovaries
    B. Metastasis of breast cancer to axillary nodes
    C. The sudden appearance of multiple Seborrhoeic keratoses. Indicator of internal malignancy
    D. The sudden metastasis of bowel cancer to the peritoneum

Paper 2 Answers

Question 1
Correct Answer: A

Topical ketoconazole has no place in the treatment of vitiligo; it is used in treating fungal infections. Topical corticosteroid in some may stop the enlargement/growth of patches of vitiligo. Tacrolimus and Pimecrolimus are alternatives to steroid cream, that may also work in preventing the spread/enlargement. Topical ketoconazole has no place in the treatment of vitiligo; it is used in treating fungal infections. It must be noted that there is no cure for vitiligo. Some patients may use skin camouflage creams to cover the white patches. Narrow UVB band therapy may also be indicated in the treatment of vitiligo. Sunblock is advised if patients wish to prevent an increased difference in colour between their original skin tone and areas affected by vitiligo. However, if vitiligo doesn't bother an individual, then there is no need for treatment.

Question 2
Correct Answer: A

This gentleman has alopecia areata, specifically patchy alopecia. Patchy alopecia is the most common type, with localised areas of hair loss. Extensive alopecia is where >50% of hair is lost. Alopecia totalis means all scalp hair is lost. Alopecia universalis is the complete loss of all body hair. Alopecia areata is a condition where there are patches of hair loss. "Exclamation marks" are characteristic of this condition. Apart from this, the scalp will look healthy and normal.

Question 3
Correct Answer: B

Porphyrias are a group of metabolic conditions where there is a problem in the production of haem. In red blood cells, haem is used to make haemoglobin. Haem is mainly produced in the liver and bone marrow.

In total, there are seven types of porphyrias, and typically they are inherited. For every kind, there is a lack of a type of **enzyme** which means that all the steps in the haem synthesis can't be completed. Therefore, there is a build-up of substances that are made during the process of haem synthesis, e.g., porphyrins. It is the build-up of these substances that causes symptoms in porphyrias.

Question 4
Correct Answer: A

Most porphyrias are autosomal dominant; however, porphyria cutanea tarda is the exception because sometimes occurs with no family history there is no family history of it. In this case, it may be triggered by alcohol and some medications.

Question 5
Correct Answer: C

Acute intermittent a porphyria is a severe form of porphyria due to a deficiency in porphobilinogen deaminase (PBGD). In Erythropoietic protoporphyria, the ferrochelatase enzyme is deficient. In porphyria cutanea tarda, there is a lack of uroporphyrinogen decarboxylase (UROD). It is the most common porphyria worldwide. Answer D is not an enzyme but the substance that builds up in excess in Erythropoietic protoporphyria.

Question 6
Correct Answer: C

In erythropoietic protoporphyria, due to a deficiency in the ferrochelatase enzyme, there is an excess of protoporphyrin. Below is a table listing the three main types of porphyrias, their deficient enzyme and the excess substrate due to this deficiency.

	Acute intermittent porphyria	Porphyria cutanea tarda	Erythropoietic protoporphyria
Enzyme deficiency	Porphobilinogen deaminase	Uroporphyrinogen decarboxylase (UROD)	Ferrochelatase
Buildup of	Porphobilinogen	Uroporphyrinogen III	Protoporphyrin

Question 7
Correct Answer: C

In erythropoietic protoporphyria, the symptoms are normally noticed in childhood. On exposure to sunlight there is burning, redness and itching on the skin. Typically, there is no blistering or scarring. Liver failure may occur due to build-up of porphyrins and other precursors. In porphyria cutanea tarda, symptoms usually develop in the patient's 40s. On exposure to sunlight, the patient's skin will appear red and blister. The skin may be fragile, itchy, hyperpigmented, and there may be hypertrichosis and milia. The urine may turn red (due to increased renal excretion of porphyrins). In acute intermittent porphyria, the symptoms usually come in waves and periods in between where the patient is symptom free. An attack may be triggered by a variety of things, e.g., medications, smoking, alcohol, emotional upset and pregnancy. The most common symptom is severe abdominal pain. There may also be constipation, nausea, vomiting and urinary tract issues. Weakness and numbness are often experienced by patients due to the nervous system being affected. Furthermore, it can affect a patient's mental health, including mania, depression, hallucinations and agitation.

Question 8

Correct Answer: B

Notably, most people affected by porphyria cutanea tarda have no family history.

Question 9
Correct Answer: A

In acute intermittent porphyria, there is an autosomal dominant genetic mutation in the HMBS gene. In erythropoietic protoporphyria, there is a genetic mutation in the FECH gene that codes for the production of ferrochelatase. Commonly patients with porphyria cutanea tarda have no family history of porphyrias.

Question 10
Correct Answer: B

Tuberous sclerosis is a genetic condition causing the formation of hamartomas, including on the brain, skin and kidneys. The mutation is either in the TSC1 gene on chromosome 9 - responsible for the production of hamartin or a mutation in the TSC2 gene on chromosome 16 - responsible for the production of tuberin. Neurofibromatosis type 1 is an autosomal dominant genetic disorder, with a mutation of the NF1 gene on chromosome 17. Gorlin's syndrome is an autosomal dominant condition that is due to a mutation in the PTCH1 gene on chromosome 9. It is a genetic condition where an individual has multiple basal cell carcinomas. Wilson's disease is an autosomal recessive condition characterised by excess copper in the body. The defect is located on chromosome 13.

Question 11
Correct Answer: A

Tuberous sclerosis normally presents as autosomal dominant.
Question 12

Correct Answer: D

Neurofibromatosis type 1, also known as Von Recklinghausen's syndrome, is characterised by café-au-lait spots, axillary or inguinal freckles, Lisch nodules (hamartomas of the iris), neurofibromas or plexiform neurofibroma and optic nerve gliomas. Diagnosis is via genetic testing.

Question 13
Correct Answer: A

Tuberous sclerosis is characterised by subungual fibromas (skin-coloured tumours in the nail folds), facial angiofibromas, ash-leaf macules (fluoresce under UV light), shagreen patches (roughened patches of skin over the lumbar spine) and adenoma sebaceum (angiofibromas) in a butterfly distribution over the nose. Epilepsy and developmental features are associated with this condition too. Ash-leaf macules are normally the earliest cutaneous sign. Neurofibromatosis type 2 is a condition associated with bilateral vestibular schwannomas and meningiomas. Psoriasis, specifically, psoriatic arthritis is associated with nail abnormalities such as pitting, onycholysis and subungual hyperkeratosis, however, subungual fibromas are not seen. In psoriatic arthritis, a "pencil in the cup" is characteristic on an x-ray.

Question 14
Correct Answer: B

Xeroderma pigmentosum is a rare, autosomal recessive disorder where there is a problem with the skin's ability to repair DNA damage from ultraviolet (UV) light. This results in photosensitivity, higher incidence of cancer at a very young age, xerosis, poikiloderma (areas of hypopigmentation, hyper-pigmentation, telangiectasia and atrophy). Eyes features include photophobia, conjunctival inflammation and keratitis and tumours of conjunctiva and eyelids.

Gorlin's syndrome is a genetic condition that should be suspected in younger people with basal cell carcinomas. Other features include pitting of palms and soles, jaw cysts, spine and rib anomalies, calcification of falx cerebri and cataracts. Epidermolysis bullosa is a genetic condition characterised by skin fragility and blistering of the skin. Albinism is a genetic condition in which patients produce little/no melanin pigment. Features include marked reduction in the colour of the skin, hair and eyes, easily sunburned and numerous eye problems, e.g., impaired vision, photophobia and nystagmus.

Question 15
Correct Answer: B

In Xeroderma pigmentosum there is a mutation in the NER genes. Normal functioning NER genes are responsible for removing abnormal sections of DNA as a result of sun damage. Genetic mutations in these genes produce a build-up of abnormal genetic material, promoting the growth of skin cancers.

Question 16
Correct Answer: C

Part of skin	Embryological origin
Epidermis	Ectoderm
Dermis	Mesoderm
Melanocytes	Neural crest

Question 17
Correct Answer: A

The Blaschko lines are the lines of normal skin development. They do not follow a pattern of nerves, vessels or lymphatics.

Question 18

Correct Answer: B

Stratum granulosum (granular layer) contains Odland bodies.
Below is a table listing the Latin equivalent of the layers of the epidermis:

Layers of the epidermis	Latin equivalent
Keratin layer	Stratum corneum
Granular layer	Stratum granulosum
Prickle cell layer	Stratum spinosum
Basal cell layer	Stratum basale

Question 19
Correct Answer: D

There are two main types of melanin. Firstly, eumelanin which is a darker pigment that predominates in black and brunette hair. Secondly, phaeomelanin, which is a lighter pigment found in red hair. Melanocytes move melanin into small sacs called melanosomes, and they convert tyrosine into the melanin pigment. Melanocytes are pigment-producing dendritic cells. They are found in the basal layer and above.

Question 20
Correct Answer: A

Condition	Problem with melanocytes
Albinism	Partial loss of pigment production
Vitiligo	Autoimmune disease with loss of melanocytes
Malignant melanoma	Tumour of melanocytes

Nelson's syndrome	Melanin stimulating hormone is produced in excess in the pituitary gland, post bilateral adrenalectomy for Cushing's syndrome.

Question 21
Correct Answer: B

Merkel cells are mechanoreceptors that respond to a light-touch vibration. They are found within the basal layer, between keratinocytes and nerve fibres.

Question 22
Correct Answer: C

Langerhans cells are dendritic cells (antigen-presenting cells) that are contained within the prickle cell layer of the epidermis. They are also found in the dermis and lymph nodes. These cells originate in the bone marrow. Langerhans cells contain Birbeck granules that look like tennis racquets on histology.

Question 23
Correct Answer: B

Apocrine glands are found in the axillae, pubic area, anus and nipple area.

There are three types of skin glands. Namely:

Name of skin gland	Location of skin gland	Function	Extra information
Sebaceous	Chest, back, scalp, face and forehead	Secretes oily substance (sebum) that moisturises the skin (skin lubrication and protection from fungal infection.	Clinically relevant for acne and folliculitis.

Apocrine	Axillae, pubic area, anus and nipple area	Secretes sweat. Secretions contain more lipids and proteins than eccrine, and the bacteria feed off this, leading to the production of bad smell (odour).	These sweat glands are androgen-dependent and therefore develop during puberty.
Eccrine glands	Found all over the body but in particular the soles of feet, palms of hands, axillae and forehead. Not found on the lips or genitals.	Main active sweat gland. Involved in cooling by evaporation (therefore may have a role in temperature regulation) and moistens palms/soles to aid grip.	Eccrine glands are the most common gland on the face. There is a sympathetic supply.

Question 24
Correct Answer: A

The pilosebaceous unit consists of hair, hair follicle, sebaceous gland and the arrector pili muscle.

Question 25
Correct Answer: C

Stage of the hair growth	What occurs in the stage	Length of the stage
Anagen	Growing phase	3-7 years
Catagen	Involuting phase	3-4 weeks
Telogen	Resting phase	3-6 months

A useful way to remember the order of the stages of hair growth is thinking alphabetically. E.g., Anagen, Catagen, Telogen (A -> C -> T).

Question 26
Correct Answer: B

Telogen Effluvium is characterised by hair thinning in the telogen phase.

Condition	Description
Alopecia Areata	An autoimmune disorder characterised by hair loss (classic exam description is "examination marks"). Hair loss occurs in small patches.
Telogen Effluvium	Hair loss after stress/trauma/pregnancy. It is characterised by a hair thinning in the telogen phase.
Androgenic Alopecia	A genetic condition that affects both men and women. Men - called male pattern baldness, can begin in teens or early 20s. It is characterised by a receding hairline and a gradual disappearance of hair from the frontal scalp and crown. Women - called female pattern baldness. Typically, doesn't occur till 40 years or later—usually general thinning of the entire cap, most noticeably at the crown.
Hirsutism	Hirsutism is excess hair in men and a male pattern of hair distribution in women.
Virilisation	When a woman develops a male growth pattern and other masculine physical traits, this can occur due to excess androgen from a tumour.

Question 27
Correct Answer: A

Meissner's corpuscles detect vibration and fine touch.

The skin contains an autonomic nerve supply for the blood vessels, nerves and glands. However, it also has somatic sensory (dermatomes) - containing two types of nerves.
1. Free nerve endings - pain
2. Special receptors: Pacinian corpuscles which detect pressure and Meissner's corpuscles which detect vibration and fine touch.

Useful tip: to remember the difference between the special receptors is Pacinian begins with P and therefore is associated with pressure.

Question 28
Correct Answer: D

Keratinocytes are responsible for vitamin D metabolism. Below are different parts/features of the skin and their functions within the skin.

Part/feature of skin	Function
Blood vessels	Temperature regulation, nutrition and oxygenation
Fibroblast	Collagen synthesis
Keratin layer	Waterproof barrier
Melanocytes	DNA protection from ultraviolet light
Sebaceous gland	Skin lubrication
Keratinocyte	Vitamin D metabolism
Subcutaneous fat	Energy storage
Collagen	Tensile strength
Basal cells	Epidermal proliferation
Eccrine glands	Moistens palms/soles for grip
Sebaceous glands	Maintains skin barrier
Meissner's corpuscles	Vibration and fine touch sensation
Lymphatics	Immune surveillance
Apocrine glands	Scent glands
Pacinian corpuscles	Pressure sensation

Question 29
Correct Answer: B

A patient that usually burns and sometimes tans is type II on the Fitzpatrick scale.

The Fitzpatrick scale is a classification based on an individual's skin colour and their response to ultraviolet (UV) light. In the skin, the quantity of melanin pigment produced by melanocytes determines how a patient responds on exposure to UV light.

The number on the Fitzpatrick scale	Skin colour	Response to ultraviolet light
I	Very pale white skin. Blonde or red hair. Blue or green eyes.	Always burns, cannot tan.
II	Pale white/fair skin. Blue or green eyes.	Usually burns, sometimes tans.
III	Darker white skin	Sometimes burns usually tans. The burn will turn to tan.
IV	Olive/light brown	Burns minimally tans easily.
V	Brown	Very rarely burns, tans very easily.
VI	Black or dark brown	Never burns, always tans.

Question 30
Correct Answer: A

Urticaria, angioedema, atopy (e.g., asthma, eczema and hayfever) are all type 1 hypersensitivity reactions. These are IgE antibody-mediated immune responses, following exposure to a specific antigen.

Hypersensitivity describes an overreaction/exaggeration of the normal immune response to an antigen. There are four types of hypersensitivity reactions. These are categorised depending on immunological involvement and the time frame of the response. They are listed below:

Hypersensitivity Type	Description	Conditions following this hypersensitivity type
1	Immediate - IgE mediated	Urticaria, Angioedema, Atopy (e.g., asthma, eczema and rhinitis)
2	Antibody - IgG, IgM	Pemphigus Vulgaris, Bullous Pemphigoid
3	Complement mediated	Most autoimmune conditions, e.g., Systemic lupus erythematous
4	Delayed - Cell-mediated Th1 cells	Allergic contact dermatitis, Scabies

Allergy is a hypersensitivity disorder causing an exaggerated immune response to a normally harmless substance in the environment.

Question 31
Correct Answer: C

The hyponychium is the underlying free edge of the nail plate. Answers A, B and D are all incorrect. The growth rate of fingernails is quicker than toenails. Also, toe and fingernails grow faster in the summer than the winter. The cuticle of the nail is an extension of the skin fold, covering the nail root. The nail plate sits on the nail bed.

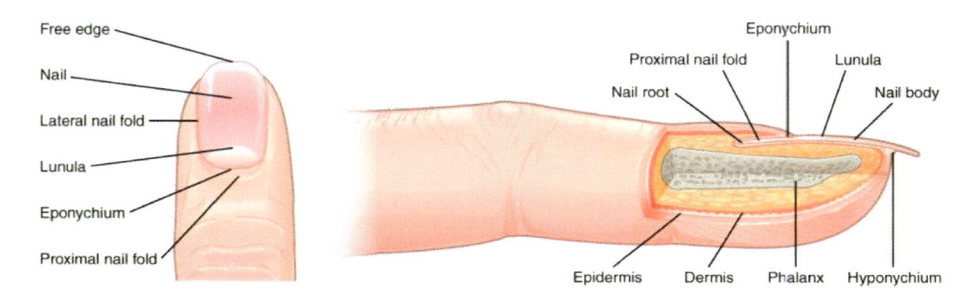

Question 32
Correct Answer: A and C

Psoriasis is associated with TH1 and TH17.

Immunological cell	Associated Condition
TH1	Psoriasis
TH2	Atopic dermatitis
TH17	Psoriasis and atopic dermatitis

Question 33
Correct Answer: C

Immunological cell	Function
CD8+ cytotoxic T cells	Protect against viruses and cancer
CD4+ helper T cells	TH1 cells activate macrophages to destroy microorganisms. TH2 cells help B cells to make antibodies.
B cells	Secrete antibodies (part of the humoral response)

Question 34
Correct Answer: B

MHC class 2 are found on antigen-presenting cells (B cells and macrophages) and present to T helper cells (CD4+ cells). MHC class 1 is located on almost all cells and presents antigens to cytotoxic T cells (CD8+ T cells). The major histocompatibility complex (MHC) is a set of genes that code for proteins on the cell surface. These are needed for the acquired immune system to recognise foreign molecules/cells. MHC is found on the short arm of chromosome 6. MHC is responsible for organ transplant rejection

Question 35
Correct Answer: D

"Enables the organism to avoid host defence mechanisms" best describes Impedin. Virulence factors of bacteria are molecules produced by bacteria that add to their effectiveness and enable them to replicate and disseminate within a host.

Virulence factors of bacteria:

Virulence factors of bacteria	Description
Adhesion	Enables the binding of the organism to the host tissue.
Invasin	Enables the organism to invade a host cell/tissue
Impedin	Enables the organism to avoid the host defence mechanisms.
Aggressin	This causes damage to the host directly.
Modulin	This induces damage to the host indirectly.

Question 36
Correct Answer: A

A cream is "a semisolid emulsion of oil in water; it contains an emulsifier and preservative".

Question 37
Correct Answer: B

Ointments are more suitable for very dry or hyperkeratotic areas. A vehicle is a substance, without any therapeutic action, that is used in combination with a drug to aid administration. Examples of some are listed in the table below:

Types of vehicles	Description	Use

Creams	Semisolid emulsion of oil in water.	Contain an emulsifier and preservative. Non-greasy. Moisturiser. Note: more likely to cause skin sensitisation due to containing preservatives. They are used in the treatment of many conditions, e.g., eczema, allergies, insect bites.
Ointments	A semisolid grease/oil.	No preservative. Greasy. Occlusive/restrict trans epidermal water loss. Better for very dry or hyperkeratotic areas.
Lotion	A suspension/solution of a drug in either water, alcohol or another form of liquid.	It is used for the scalp, hair-bearing areas. Possibility of stinging/dry skin if contains alcohol.
Gels	Thickened aqueous lotions. Gels are semisolids containing high molecular weight polymers, e.g., methylcellulose.	It is cosmetically acceptable. They are used for the scalp, hair-bearing areas and face.
Paste	Finely powdered material, forming a semisolid.	Greasy, stiff, protective, occlusive and hydration. They are used for under bandages.
Foams	The hydrophilic liquid in continuous phase with **foaming agent dispersed in gas.**	Spreads easily over large areas. Not greasy. Increases penetration of active agents, e.g., steroid, vitamin D

Question 38
Correct Answer: A

A "stuck on appearance" best describes a basal cell papilloma (Seborrhoeic keratoses). Basal cell carcinoma is a translucent or pearly nodule with telangiectasia and with rolled raised edges. In the exams, it is often described as "picket fence pearly border, rodent ulcer". Squamous cell carcinoma presents as a hyperkeratotic lesion with crusting and ulceration. Acne vulgaris consists of papules, comedones, pustules, nodules and cysts.

Question 39
Correct Answer: A

This teenager is having a type I hypersensitivity reaction. The patient is in anaphylaxis, with low blood pressure and airway swelling, highlighted by the bilateral respiratory wheeze. Type 1 hypersensitivity occurs within minutes to hours, and the patient can experience urticaria, pruritus, erythema, angioedema and anaphylaxis. In a type II hypersensitivity reaction, the patient typically has a past medical history or a family history of autoimmune disease. Type III reactions aren't necessary to know for dermatology at this level. Type IV hypersensitivity reactions are also known as allergic contact dermatitis. These are delayed, abnormal T-cell mediated immune responses to a specific antigen, e.g., to latex or nickel.

Question 40
Correct Answer: D

This patient has allergic contact dermatitis (type IV hypersensitivity reaction), which is commonly caused by nickel, a component of some watches. Type IV is a delayed response and presents typically 12-72 hours from the initial exposure.
Typically, there is a rash and pruritus. It is essential not to be confused with irritant dermatitis because this is not immune-mediated and occurs due to repeated contact with irritant substances on normal skins

Question 41
Correct Answer: B

Diagnosis of a type IV hypersensitivity reactions is made with patch testing – this involves the testing of common or suspected allergens to the patient. Answers A, C and D are all used in the diagnosis of type I hypersensitivity reactions.

Question 42
Correct Answer: B

This patient has Lichen planus, which presents as an itchy rash. Found most commonly on the soles, palms, genitalia and flexor surfaces of the arms. Eczema is characterised by dry, itchy and erythematous skin. Most commonly affecting the hands and the flexural surface of the elbows. In children, it is seen most commonly on the face and scalp. Psoriasis is most widely seen on the extensor surfaces and causes scaly skin, with erythematous itchy skin. Pityriasis alba is a self-limiting condition that causes fine-scaled, dry and pale patches on the patient's face.

Question 43
Correct Answer: D

Propionibacterium acnes is the bacteria that is relevant in acne. *Propionibacterium acnes* infection secretes lipases causing inflammation and the breakdown of sebum. Overall causing pustule formation. *Staphylococcus aureus* and *Staphylococcus epidermidis* are found as commensals on the outer layer of the skin.

Question 44
Correct Answer: D

Acanthosis nigricans is a skin discolouration characterised by a darkening of the skin, especially at the folds of the skin, e.g., axilla, neck and groin. It is most commonly associated with malignancy, especially GI adenocarcinoma or type 2 diabetes.

Question 45
Correct Answer: C

Leser-Trélat sign is a sudden appearance of multiple Seborrhoeic keratoses. This is an indicator of gastrointestinal tract carcinoma.

Paper 3 Questions

1. Which diagnosis is most likely in a patient presenting with pruritic papules involving the extensor surfaces of his elbows and knees?

A.	Dermatitis Herpetiformis
B.	Henoch-Schonlein Purpura (HSP)
C.	Diabetes
D.	Idiopathic thrombocytopenic purpura

2. A 30-year-old female presented with bilateral erythematous skin lesions on her shins. On examination, her skin has a shiny orange peel quality.

What is this a sign of?

A.	Pretibial myxoedema
B.	Erythema Nodosum
C.	Pyoderma gangrenosum
D.	Necrobiosis lipoidica

3. A 50-year-old female (with underlying inflammatory bowel disease) presented with a small red papule that later developed into a large painful, necrotic ulcer with a violaceus border.

What is the likely diagnosis?

A.	Pretibial myxoedema

B. Erythema Nodosum
C. Pyoderma gangrenosum
D. Necrobiosis lipoidica

4. A patient escapes a house fire in the middle of the night. Whilst examining him, you note parts of his skin appear white and others appear black. There are no blisters visible. The patient reports very little sensation on the affected parts of his skin.

What degree of burn does he have?

A. Dermal
B. Superficial dermal
C. Full Thickness
D. 4th degree burn

5. A 5-year-old boy presents with a golden crusty lesion around the lips.

What is the likely pathogen?

A. Herpes simplex
B. Coxsackievirus A16
C. Staphylococcus aureus
D. Staphylococcus epidermidis

6. A 60-year-old lady presented with a superficial, red, erythematous lesion of 10cm diameter on her right leg. She reported it was only about 3cm a few hours ago. On examination the area is hot, tender and red. The patient has also developed a low-grade fever. Her other leg is unaffected.

What is the likely diagnosis?

A. Venous Eczema
B. Cellulitis
C. Necrotising fasciitis
D. Gas Gangrene

7. A dog walker presents with fever, sore throat, and painful knees. On examination, a bulls' eye rash is seen on the patient's leg which she states developed 4 days after a walk in the fields. The patient is systemically well.

What is the likely diagnosis?

A. Septic arthritis
B. Lyme disease
C. Influenza infection
D. Lupus

8. A 15-year-old boy develops a sore throat and fever. On examination there is exudative tonsillitis, a strawberry tongue and sandpaper rash on his body.

What is the likely diagnosis?

A. Kawasaki's disease
B. Viral Tonsillitis
C. Measles
D. Scarlet fever

9. A 22-year-old university student presents to his GP with severe itching in his hands, wrists and axillae which is worse at night. On examination you find linear vesicular lesions in the interdigital web spaces in his hands. He mentions his flat mates are also complaining of itching.

What is the treatment for this condition?

A. Permethrin cream 5% applied twice one week apart only for him
B. Permethrin cream 5% once off for him and his flat mates
C. Permethrin cream 5% once off only for him
D. Permethrin cream 5% applied twice, one week apart for him and his flat mates

10. A 6-year-old girl presents with intense itching of her scalp particularly behind the ears and the nape of the neck. A few of her classmates have the same problem. On examination, there are red brown spots visible on the scalp.

Which of the following is not appropriate?

A. Treat family members with Malathion cream
B. Keep home from school
C. Inform school
D. Use of Nit coombs on wet hair

11. A 6-year-old boy complains of itching in his anus which he says is much worse at night. He is otherwise well and there is no medical history. On examination, a thin white 1cm long thread is visible in the anus. The patient is diagnosed as having threadworms, what is the correct management?

A. Mebendazole
B. Metronidazole
C. Amoxicillin
D. Clotrimazole

12. A 70-year-old lady has multiple pigmented raised papules on her back. Her husband says they have been there for a few years. On examination you see multiple small brown to dark lesions that have a characteristic stuck on appearance.

What is the likely diagnosis?

A. Basal cell carcinoma
B. Basal cell papilloma
C. Melanocytic naevi
D. Squamous cell carcinoma

13. Which one of the following is not a feature of an atypical melanocytic naevus?

A. Poorly defined margins
B. Evenly pigmented
C. >5mm in size
D. Asymmetry

14. A 20-year-old patient visits her GP complaining of multiple telangiectasia on her lips. She admits to a lifelong history of recurrent nose bleeds and minor rectal bleeds. She mentions that her mum also has recurrent nose bleeds.

What is the likely diagnosis?

A. Hereditary haemorrhagic telangiectasia (HHT)
B. Limited systemic sclerosis (Crest syndrome)
C. Von Willebrand disease (VWb)
D. Haemophilia

15. An elderly lady with a background of diabetes complains of an enlarging ulcer on her distal left leg. On examination, the ulcer lies above the medial malleolus, with surrounding haemosiderin staining and significant lipodermatosclerosis of the skin. There are also marked varicose veins.

What is the likely diagnosis?

A. Neuropathic ulcer
B. Arterial leg ulcer
C. Venous leg ulcer
D. Chronic leg ischaemia

16. An elderly lady comes to your dermatology clinic with a painful leg ulcer. Her ABPI is 0.43. Clinically the ulcer does not appear infected.

Which of the following treatment options is the most appropriate?

A. Full graduated compression bandage
B. Reduced compression bandage
C. Refer to vascular surgeons
D. Take a swab of the ulcer and ask the patient to come back after the results.

17. An elderly lady comes to your dermatology clinic with a leg ulcer. Her ABPI is 0.7. The ulcer is not painful and there are no features suggestive of infection.

Which of the following treatment options is the most appropriate?

A. Full graduated compression bandage
B. Reduced compression bandage
C. Refer to vascular surgeons
D. Take a swab of the ulcer and ask the patient to come back after the results.

18. A patient suffers a cut on the tips of their fingers. A few days later, they develop a raised purplish lesion at the same site of injury which bleeds profusely with contact.

What is the likely diagnosis?

A. Pyogenic granuloma
B. Kaposi sarcoma
C. Abscess
D. Haemangioma

19. A red collection of spots in a butterfly distribution on the face is associated with which feature of tuberous sclerosis?

A. Adenoma sebaceum
B. Koenen's tumours
C. Ash leaf spots
D. Shagreen patches

20. A 30-year-old female presented with bilateral tender nodules on her shins with surrounding erythema. She is otherwise fit and well and the only medication she takes is the combined oral contraceptive pill.

What is the likely sign?

A. Pretibial myxoedema
B. Erythema nodosum
C. Pyoderma gangrenosum
D. Necrobiosis lipoidica

21. Which of the following is the most likely diagnosis in a child presenting with abdominal discomfort and palpable purpuric, non-pruritic lesions of the extensor surfaces of his elbows and knees?

A. Dermatitis herpetiformis
B. Henoch-Schonlein Purpura (HSP)
C. Diabetes
D. Idiopathic thrombocytopenic purpura

22. Which of the following statements about basal cell carcinoma (BCC) is true?

A. Usually develop on photo-protected sites
B. Commonly affect darker skin types (Fitzpatrick phototype 5-6)
C. Spread via local invasion
D. Rapidly enlarge over days to weeks

23. A 40-year-old patient with a history of chronic alcohol excess presents with an erythematous, scaly rash on her face. She also complains of severe diarrhoea and abdominal pain. Her husband mentions she is increasingly forgetful and sometimes complains that she is now seeing things that are not there.

What vitamin deficiency is this presentation likely due to?

A. Vitamin A deficiency
B. Vitamin B1 deficiency
C. Vitamin B3 deficiency
D. Vitamin B12 deficiency

24. A patient has a sternotomy scar following a recent open-heart surgery. She later develops a painful, firm hard growth that extends beyond the original wound.

What is the likely diagnosis?

A. Keloid scar
B. Hypertrophic scar
C. Basal cell carcinoma
D. Dermatofibrosarcoma

25. An 8-year-old boy presents with a 5-day fever that is unresponsive to regular paracetamol. On examination, you noticed bilateral conjunctivitis, a strawberry tongue and a shedding rash of the extremities.

Which of the following investigations is most important to request?

A. Blood cultures
B. Autoimmune screen
C. LFT's
D. Echocardiogram

26. A 15-year-old girl presents to her GP with multiple comedones, papules and pustules on her face, back and chest. There are no nodules, inflammatory lesions or scarring. She has tried topical benzoyl peroxide with no effect and feels the lesions are worsening.

What is the next most appropriate step in her management?

A. Topical doxycycline
B. Oral erythromycin
C. Oral lymecycline
D. Oral isotretinoin

27. A 35-year-old lady complains of recurrent episodes of facial flushing, erythema and pustules on her face. There is associated telangiectasia. She complains that alcohol makes her rash worse.

What is the likely diagnosis?

A. Chronic alcoholism
B. Acne rosacea
C. Hereditary haemorrhagic telangiectasia
D. Seborrhoeic dermatitis

28. A 30-year-old man presents with inflamed greasy skin affecting his face, with a focus of scale around his eyebrows and nasolabial area. He also suffers from dandruff.

What is the likely diagnosis?

A. Contact irritant dermatitis
B. Allergic dermatitis
C. Acne rosacea
D. Seborrhoeic dermatitis

29. A patient escapes a house fire in the middle of the night. He suffers full thickness burns covering 50% of his skin and is admitted to ITU. On discharge, he complains of severe epigastric pain.

What is the likely diagnosis?

A. Perforated duodenal ulcer
B. Cushing ulcer
C. H. pylori
D. Curling ulcer

30. A 30-year-old diabetic female presented with a painless shiny yellow-red skin discolouration with associated telangiectasia.

What is the likely sign?

A. Pretibial myxoedema
B. Erythema nodosum
C. Pyoderma gangrenosum
D. Necrobiosis lipoidica

31. Which hypersensitivity is associated with acute urticaria due to food allergy?

A. Type 1
B. Type 2
C. Type 3
D. Type 4

32. An 8-year-old boy presents with abdominal pain and joints pains. He later develops a purpuric rash down his buttocks and thighs and feels unwell.

Which of the following initial investigations should always be considered?

A. Anti-transglutaminase antibodies (anti-tTg)
B. Abdominal X-ray
C. Urinalysis and U&Es
D. Lumbar Puncture

33. A skin biopsy was performed on a patient in your dermatology clinic. The report states there is an absent granular layer with evidence of hyperproliferation of keratinocytes.

What condition is this histopathological description in keeping with?

A. Lichen planus
B. Psoriasis
C. Pemphigus vulgaris
D. Dermatitis

34. A patient presents with a non-healing leg ulcer. Her ABPI is greater than 0.8.

Which of the following is a suitable management?

A. Full graduated compression bandage
B. Reduced compression bandage
C. TED stockings
D. Wound dressings

35. A 5-year-old boy presents with a golden crusty rash on his face. You decide to investigate.

What is the most appropriate investigation?

A. Viral swab
B. FBC and CRP
C. Bacterial swab
D. Blood cultures

36. Which of the following statements best fits with bullous pemphigoid?

A. Linear IgG and C3 bands at the dermo-epidermal junction
B. IgG and C3 at the epidermis

C. IgA in the dermis
D. Granular basement membrane IgG

37. A 20-year-old girl develops blisters on her top lip which are painful, and itchy. It goes away after 5 days. She mentions this problem has occurred multiple times and would like a test to find out what it could be.

What test could you offer next this time this occurs?

A. Autoantibody screen for autoimmune diseases
B. Viral swab
C. Skin scrapes
D. Bacterial swap

38. Which of the following statements about pemphigus vulgaris is false?

A. Due to antibodies against desmoglein 3
B. There is rarely mucosal involvement
C. Nikolsky's sign is positive
D. Clinically, it presents with superficial fluid filled blisters that easily rupture

39. A patient complains of redness, itching, and scaling at the site of their new ring that they have been wearing for the past few weeks.

What is the likely diagnosis?

A. Contact irritant dermatitis
B. Atopic Dermatitis
C. Contact allergic dermatitis
D. Chronic actinic dermatitis

40. A 22-year-old foundation year one doctor started washing his hands with soap after every patient contact, after the COVID-19 outbreak. He complains that his hands are now dry, erythematous and uncomfortable.

What is the likely diagnosis?

A. Contact irritant dermatitis

B. Atopic dermatitis
C. Contact allergic dermatitis
D. Chronic actinic dermatitis

41. A 40-year-old obese female, on the contraceptive pill, with a family history of gallstones presents with acute abdominal pain which radiates to the back. On examination, you find bilateral flank ecchymosis.

What is this referred as?

A. Cullen Sign
B. Gray Turner's sign
C. Pemphigoid gestationis
D. Erythema multiforme

42. A 16-year-old boy complains of itchy sensation between his toes. On examination, you notice white scaling and flaking.

Which of the following is not an appropriate first line treatment?

A. Topical terbinafine
B. Topical nystatin
C. Topical betnovate
D. Topical miconazole

43. A 5-year-old girl presents with a dry itchy rash in the flexural surfaces of her elbows, and behind her knees. This is usually worse in the summer.

What is the likely diagnosis?

A. Contact irritant dermatitis
B. Atopic dermatitis
C. Contact allergic dermatitis
D. Chronic actinic dermatitis

44. A 25-year-old hairdresser complains of sore, itchy, dry hands. This usually improves when she is not at work. She wonders if there is any test that could be done to investigate the problem.

A. Radioallergosorbent test (RAST)
B. Skin biopsy
C. Skin prick test
D. Patch Test

45. A mother brings her 4-week-old to your surgery as she has noticed multiple small white papules around the nose and the eyes, present since birth. These cause no symptoms.

What is the likely diagnosis?

A. Milia
B. Folliculitis
C. Molluscum contagiosum
D. Childhood acne

Paper 3 Answers

Question 1
Correct Answer: A

Dermatitis herpetiformis is an autoimmune condition caused by deposition of IgA in the dermis. It is associated with coeliac disease and can be considered as the cutaneous manifestation of the disease.

Features:
- Intensely pruritic, papular rash which may be vesicular, typically found on extensor surfaces, in particular, the elbows, knees, buttocks. Can also occur on the abdomen.
- Biopsy: direct immunofluorescence reveals IgA deposition in the dermis.

Diagnosis of Coeliac disease:
- Initial test: IgA anti-tissue transglutaminase antibody

- Diagnostic test: duodenal biopsy showing villous atrophy

Management:
- Gluten free diet

Question 2
Correct Answer: A

Pretibial myxoedema is localised thickening of the skin due to diffuse accumulation of glycosaminoglycans in the dermis and subcutaneous tissue of the skin. It is associated with Graves' disease and may be present before clinical symptoms of the disease. It is characterised by symmetrical erythematous skin lesions often described as shiny, orange peel skin. It may also present as localised non-pitting oedema.

Question 3
Correct Answer: C

Pyoderma gangrenosum (PG) is an inflammatory skin disease known as neutrophilic dermatoses and is the second most common cutaneous manifestation of IBD.
Most commonly, PG is idiopathic. It can arise after sustaining minor injury/trauma (a phenomenon called pathergy). It is characterised by a red small papule, that often rapidly progresses into a very painful large necrotic ulcer with a characteristic violaceous edge.

Question 4
Correct Answer: C

A burn is an injury caused by thermal, chemical, electrical or radiation energy.

Degree of burn:

- Epidermal (superficial partial thickness): red, painful, no blistering.
- Superficial dermal: Pale pink, mottled skin with small blisters
- Dermal: Cherry red, blistering, reduced sensation.
- Full thickness (previously third degree): White or black, no blisters, absent sensation. Requires grafting.
- Fourth Degree: Involves subcutaneous fat, muscle and even bone.

Complications:
- Hypovolemic shock
- Haemolysis
- Secondary infection
- Peptic ulcer (called a curling ulcer)

Question 5
Correct Answer: C

This patient has presented with signs of impetigo. Impetigo is a superficial bacterial skin infection most commonly caused by staphylococcus aureus or streptococcus pyogenes (Group-A Streptococcus).

Features:
- Golden crusty erosions are seen most commonly on the face but can also affect limbs and flexures.
- Commonly affects pre-school children. The child is usually well but due to the highly infectious nature of impetigo, avoid contact with other children till the crusts clear.

Management:
- Regular washing of the areas to remove the crust
- Topical fusidic acid for localised infection, though high risk of resistance
- Oral flucloxacillin for widespread infection
- Lesions are infectious until crusting occurs or 48 hours after antibiotics.

Herpes simplex causes cold sores which are painful itchy vesicles found around the mouth. Coxsackievirus A16 causes hand, foot, and mouth disease which will be covered elsewhere in the book. Staphylococcus epidermidis is a gram-positive coagulase negative bacterium that usually causes infections where there are foreign devices - such as arterial lines, PICC line. It can also cause endocarditis and endophthalmitis.

Question 6
Correct Answer: B

The answer here is cellulitis. The clue in the question is spreading erythema and a unilateral presentation with classic signs of inflammation.

Cellulitis is a spreading of inflammation in the dermis and subcutaneous tissue most commonly caused by staphylococcus aureus or streptococcus pyogenes. It is characterised by a unilateral painful erythematous swelling which can track. It can be associated with a fever and tachycardia. Treatment is usually with oral flucloxacillin unless the patient is septic in which case intravenous flucloxacillin is used.

Venous eczema usually presents bilaterally in both legs as orange-brown macular pigmentation due to haemosiderin deposition. This is often wrongly confused as bilateral cellulitis which is extremely rare.

Necrotising fasciitis (NF) and gas gangrene are types of rapidly progressive cellulitis which are more common in immunocompromised patients such as diabetics or those in ICU. Necrotising fasciitis is a necrotising infection of the dermis, subcutaneous tissue, fascia or the muscle. It is caused by bacteria which multiply and produce toxins resulting in tissue thrombosis.
There are two types. Type 1 is caused by a mixture of aerobes and anaerobes. Type 2 is caused by Group A streptococcus. Features include rapidly progressive cellulitis, pain, temperature, and an initial systemic upset out of proportion to physical signs. Management is with immediate surgical debridement and IV antibiotic therapy.

Gas gangrene is caused by clostridium perfringens. It causes rapid muscle necrosis, gas production, and severe sepsis. Gases produced include hydrogen, carbon dioxide, nitrogen and oxygen. Clinical examination would reveal crepitus in the skin. Management is with immediate surgical debridement and IV antibiotic therapy.

Question 7
Correct Answer: B

Lyme's disease is an infection caused by Borrelia burgdorferi, a spirochaete, which is transmitted to humans from an infected tick bite. Untreated, it can lead to multisystem involvement.

Features:
- Cutaneous rash at site of tick bite, called erythema migrans.
- Signs: bulls eye / target-like rash which occurs within 3-36 days of tick bite.
- Patients may be febrile or have joint pains.
- **Stage 1 disease: Localised erythema migrans within 3-36 days.**
- Stage 2 disease: flu like illness. Occurs days to months later.
- Stage 3 disease: arthritis, polyneuropathy, encephalomyelitis, psychosis, neuroborreliosis

Investigations:
Antibody to B burgdorferi using ELISA followed by immunoblot

Management:
Investigations may be normal in very early disease, hence if clinically suspected and typical rash appears after history of a tick bite, it is important to treat to prevent serious sequelae. Doxycycline 100mg BD for up to 10-14 days.
Amoxicillin 500mg TDS in children.

Question 8
Correct Answer: D

These are typical features of Scarlet fever. Scarlet fever is a notifiable disease caused by streptococcus pyogenes.

Features:
- Inflamed sore throat covered by haemorrhagic spots or exudates
- Fever, cervical lymphadenopathy
- Strawberry tongue
- Sandpaper rash

Management:
Penicillin or azithromycin if penicillin allergy. Note: Kawasaki disease typically affects children under 5 years of age and does not present with a sandpaper rash.

Question 9
Correct Answer: D
Scabies is an intensely itchy parasitic infestation of the skin caused by the Sarcoptes scabiei mite, which burrows under the top layer of the skin. Symptoms develop about 1-month post a new infection. The patient will have been infectious during this time, which is why it is important to treat patients and close contacts prophylactically.

Risk factors:
- Prolonged contact with individuals with scabies such as sexual contact
- Poor hygiene
- Residential homes
- Homelessness and poverty

Features:
- Widespread itching, worse at night.
- Erythematous vesicular/ papular lesions seen at sites of burrows.
- Areas most commonly affected include: interdigital web spaces, genitals, axillae, and wrists. Scalp is spared in adults but can be involved in babies.

Norwegian scabies:
This is infestation with thousands of mites usually in immunocompromised patients who do not generate any immune reaction to the mites and hence get heavily infected; there may be minimal or no itch. It is characterised by crusted and hyperkeratotic lesions in web spaces/ flexures. It is highly contagious and difficult to treat. Treatment involves systemic ivermectin along with topical permethrin.

Management:
Permethrin 5% dermal cream applied twice (one week apart to kill any hatched mites) to the whole body overnight. All close contacts should also be treated on the same days. Patients may notice a worsening of itch post treatment which does not mean treatment failure. Fomites (clothing, bedding) needs to be either washed at high temperature or separated in bags for up to 3 days to kill the mites.

Question 10
Correct Answer: B

Pediculosis capitis is caused by a parasite called, pediculus humanus capitis or common head lice. It feeds on human blood. The female louse can lay 50–100 eggs at a rate of 3–6 per day; the eggs hatch after 8 days. Spread is predominantly through head-to-head contact. Risk factors include female sex and anything that may increase the chance of head-to-head contact such as sharing towels, beds, hairbrushes. Patients present with intensely itchy scalp which is worse behind the ears and nape of the neck. Red-brown spots on the skin are due to excreted digested blood and nits can be seen.

Management:
Treat all members of the family at the same time. Inform the nursery or school. There is no need to stay off school. First line agent is malathion cream – must be applied twice (7-10 days apart). Nit combs used in wet hair are the most effective way of physically removing the lice and nits.

Question 11
Correct Answer: A

Enterobius vermicularis (pinworms), also known as threadworms are roundworms that live inside the intestinal tract of humans. Infestation is common amongst school children aged 5-10.

Features:
Pruritus ani (itching around the anus) is the most common symptom and is usually worse at night when the female worm comes to the surface to lay eggs. Severe infestation can cause abdominal pain, nausea and vomiting. Spread to vagina can occur in females. Pinworms can be seen by examining the anus and can appear as a white thin thread 1-2cm in length.

Management:
- Diagnosis can be confirmed by examination under microscopy (often unnecessary)
- Good hygiene, keeping fingernails short
- Single dose of Mebendazole.

Question 12
Correct Answer: B

Seborrhoeic keratosis is a benign epidermal hyperkeratotic degenerative skin lesion also known as a basal cell papilloma.

Features:
Raised papule which can usually be skin coloured or light brown to black. Typically have a "stuck on appearance".

Management:
Reassurance.
Cryosurgery, curettage or shave biopsy can be options, particularly for irritated lesions.

Question 13
Correct Answer: B

Atypical melanocytic naevi (dysplastic naevi) have the following characteristics:
- >5mm in size
- Poorly defined margins
- Uneven pigmentation.
- Asymmetry

Question 14
Correct Answer: A

HHT is an autosomal dominant condition also known as Osler-Weber-Rendu syndrome. It is characterised by telangiectasia on the skin and mucosal surfaces including the lips, oral cavity, nasal mucosae, gastrointestinal tract and hands. It can also present in other organs such as lungs, gastrointestinal tract and central nervous system.

The diagnostic criteria include, recurrent spontaneous epistaxis, multiple telengiectases, internal organ involvement, and an affected first degree relative.

Crest syndrome is characterised by calcinosis, Raynaud's phenomenon, oesophageal dysmotility, sclerodactyly and telangiectasia.

Von Willebrand disease and haemophilia also present with bleeding tendencies. Patients with VWb usually present with nosebleeds and heavier periods. Haemophilia tends to bleed into large joints such as the knee causing swelling. Neither have telangiectasia.

Question 15
Correct Answer: C

Ulcers can be venous, arterial or neuropathic. Venous ulcers are related to venous insufficiency resulting from poorly functioning valves, which lead to backpressure of blood, increased venous pressure, and a build-up of fibrin around the capillaries. Arterial ulceration is usually due to atherosclerosis and reduced circulation to the target limb. It is more common in smokers and those who have hypertensive disease. Neuropathic ulcers usually occur in diabetic patients with peripheral neuropathy. Ulceration develops around pressure points, often secondary due to repeated trauma, such as on the sole of the foot as they lack sensory awareness.

Clinical features of leg ulcer subtypes:
1. Venous ulcers
    - Typically, above medial malleolus
    - Aching (but not painful)
    - Haemosiderin staining
    - Associated lipodermatosclerosis (erythema and hardening of skin, 'champagne bottle' appearance)
    - Varicose veins
2. Arterial ulcers
    - Appear 'punched out', sharply demarked borders
    - Painful particularly when elevated (nighttime) as this reduced blood flow to the leg further
    - Associated with cold, bluish feet
    - Often loss of appendages (hair) and appearances of shiny surrounding skin
3. Neuropathic/diabetic ulcers
    - Similar to arterial ulcers but usually on pressure areas such as heels and toes.
    - Reduced sensation oi the feet.

Question 16
Correct Answer: C

Management of leg ulcers is largely based on the ankle brachial pressure index (ABPI). Normal value is between 0.9 and 1.2. Values lower than 0.9 suggest mild arterial disease; less than 0.8 suggests moderate arterial disease; and less than 0.5 suggests severe arterial disease.

ABPI assessment:
0.9-1.2: Full graduated compression bandage (4 layer)
0.5-0.8: Reduced compression bandage
<0.5: wound debridement and care, referral to vascular surgeon.

Question 17
Correct Answer: B

Management of leg ulcers is largely based on the ankle brachial pressure index (ABPI). Normal value is between 0.9 and 1.2. Values lower than 0.9 suggest mild arterial disease; less than 0.8 suggests moderate arterial disease; and less than 0.5 suggests severe arterial disease.
ABPI assessment:
0.9-1.2: Full graduated compression bandage (4 layer)
0.5-0.8: Reduced compression bandage
<0.5: wound debridement and care, referral to vascular surgeon.

Question 18
Correct Answer: A

Pyogenic granuloma, also called eruptive haemangioma. This is neither a granuloma, nor is it pyogenic, naturally causing confusion with its name. It is idiopathic but is more common with trauma and pregnancy.

Features: small red papule commonly found on fingertips, often grows rapidly over days to weeks. Bleeds profusely and easily with trauma.

Management: They can be self-limiting. Treatment options for persistent lesions include excision or curettage and cautery under local anaesthetic, cryotherapy and topical propranolol can be used in children.

Question 19
Correct Answer: A

The following are all features of Tuberous Sclerosis:
1. Adenoma sebaceum: red collection of spots in a butterfly distribution of the face
2. Koenen's tumours (ungual or periungual fibromas): fleshy tumours that grow under the nails
3. Ash leaf spots: light-coloured patches of skin caused by melanin. Best seen under Wood's lamp.
4. Shagreen patches: thick leathery flesh coloured orange peel skin, usually seen in the lower back.

Question 20
Correct Answer: B

Erythema nodosum is an inflammatory disorder affecting the subcutaneous tissues, a 'panniculitis'. It is characterised by erythematous and symmetrical tender nodules which typically affecting the shins. In many cases no trigger is identified. It can be associated with inflammatory conditions, drugs as part of a hypersensitivity reaction and infectious conditions.

Common causes:
- Inflammatory: Sarcoidosis, inflammatory bowel disease, malignancy
- Infectious: streptococcal infections
- Iatrogenic: penicillin, sulphonamides, combined contraceptive pills.

Question 21
Correct Answer: B

HSP is an IgA mediated small vessel vasculitis which usually affects children. It typically presents with a tetrad of abdominal pain, joint pain, a palpable purpuric rash and renal disease in the form of glomerular nephritis. In children this is often self-limiting, but the condition may recur. Urinalysis should be performed to assess for renal involvement.

Dermatitis herpetiformis is an immunobullous condition associated with coeliac disease. In coeliac disease, IgA antibodies are formed which target the gut as well as the skin to form this intensely itchy purpuric rash, commonly seen on extensor surfaces such as the knees, elbows and also the buttocks.

Question 22
Correct Answer: C

Basal cell carcinomas are a locally invasive skin cancer. They develop due to cumulative amounts of sun exposure and ultraviolet related damage. BCCs are commonly seen in fairer skin types. They are usually slow growing over months to years. Although they are very unlikely to metastasise, they should be treated as they can cause local destruction to important anatomical structures.
They commonly affect photo-distributed sites including high risk sites such as areas on the face (eyelids, nose, mouth, ears).

Question 23
Correct Answer: C

Pellagra is a condition caused by niacin deficiency (vitamin B3). Primary causes are due to nutritional deficiency seen in diets in developing countries. Secondary causes are typically due to malabsorption in the presence of a normal diet such as, chronic diarrhoea, inflammatory bowel disease and liver cirrhosis. Drugs such as isoniazid can also cause as it inhibits the conversion of tryptophan to vitamin B3.

Features (4 D's):

- Diarrhoea
- Dementia
- Dermatitis: brown scaly rash on sun exposed areas.
- Death

Vitamin A deficiency called xerophthalmia causes keratomalacia and blindness. Vitamin B1 deficiency (thiamine deficiency) is common in alcoholism and may lead to Wernicke's encephalopathy. Vitamin B12 deficiency leads to macrocytic anaemia and peripheral neuropathy.

Question 24
Correct Answer: A

Keloid scars appear as a firm, smooth growth (tumour like) and arise from connective tissue of scar. They may be tender but always extend beyond the dimensions of the original wound unlike hypertrophic scars. Keloids can arise anywhere in the skin but typically arise on the sternum and upper chest area. They are more commonly seen in darker skinned individuals. The current aetiology is unknown however they are thought to have a genetic predisposition.

Hypertrophic scars are a normal scar tissue formation; the area is thicker than normal skin and does not extend beyond the original wound. Initially they may be erythematous and raised but over time they become pale and flatten.

Question 25
Correct Answer: D

Kawasaki Disease is a medium vessel vasculitis which affects children.

Features
- Fever lasting more than 5 days not responsive to paracetamol.
- Shedding rash of the extremities.
- Strawberry tongue
- Conjunctivitis and uveitis.

- Management
  - Aspirin – to reduce fever and prevent thrombosis.
  - IV immunoglobulin
  - Echocardiogram – to exclude coronary artery aneurysm

Question 26
Correct Answer: C

This patient may initially have had mild acne treated with topical benzoyl peroxide, but now she has progressed to moderate acne requiring oral antibiotics as the lesions are spread out. First line antibiotics are tetracyclines.

Acne Vulgaris is a very common skin disorder which usually starts during adolescence but can persist throughout adulthood. It is characterised by obstruction of the pilosebaceous gland, with formation of a keratin plug. This results in the formation of comedones (open and closed) and pustules as sebaceous secretions build up below the keratin plug. Colonisation often occurs with the bacterium propionibacterium acne propagating the inflammation of the hair follicle.

1. Mild Acne: open and closed comedones with little inflammatory lesions. First line treatments include topical benzoyl peroxide or retinoids. Topical antibiotics are the next step in the stepwise management of mild acne and usually a topical tetracycline is used. Oral antibiotics are the next step as with moderate acne.
2. Moderate Acne: widespread lesions which are non-inflammatory with multiple pustules. Oral tetracyclines are the first line (doxycycline, oxytetracycline, lymecycline). They are contraindicated in children under 12 and pregnancy. Erythromycin can be used as an alternative instead.
3. Severe Acne: inflammatory lesions including nodules and cysts which typically scar. Treated with oral isotretinoin (teratogenic, specialist use only).

Question 27
Correct Answer: B

Acne rosacea is a chronic relapsing condition of unknown aetiology. It typically affects the nose, cheeks and forehead. Symptoms vary and patients may present with episodes of facial flushing, erythema, pustules, and papules with associated telangiectasia and rhinophyma. Ocular involvement occurs, particularly as blepharitis. Management includes conservative advice on avoiding triggers such as heat, spicy food, alcohol, high factor sunscreen and camouflage in the form of makeup. Fixed telangiectasia can be treated with laser therapy. Mild disease can be managed with topical metronidazole, topical ivermectin and topical azelaic acid. Moderate disease or those with papules or eye disease may require oral antibiotics in the form of tetracyclines as an anti-inflammatory agent. Isotretinoin can also be used for papular disease.

Question 28
Correct Answer: D

Seborrhoeic dermatitis is a chronic form of dermatitis affecting the sebaceous glands of the scalp, face and trunk and is associated with proliferation of the fungal skin commensal Malassezia furfur. Refractory seborrhoeic dermatitis should alert clinicians of an immunosuppressive state and conditions such as HIV or malignancy should be excluded. Management includes topical agents such as zinc pyrithione and ketoconazole shampoo/ cream to any affected areas. More recalcitrant disease may require topical steroids, topical tacrolimus or even courses of oral itraconazole.

Infantile features: 'cradle cap' appearance: greasy scaling of the scalp. May spread to armpits or groins. Salmon-pink patches which tend to flake or peel.

Adult features: inflamed greasy skin with scale which affects the nasolabial folds, nose, eyebrows, ear, scalp.

Question 29
Correct Answer: D

A Curling ulcer is a peptic ulcer which occurs following burns. A Cushing ulcer is a peptic ulcer due to raised intracranial pressure.

Question 30
Correct Answer: D

Necrobiosis lipoidica is a granulomatous skin disorder that often occurs in diabetic patients. It appears on the shin as a painless shiny yellow-red patch with associated telangiectasia. Minor trauma to the area can cause ulceration. Treatment is not always successful. Diabetes should be considered as an associated condition and treatment optimised.
Topical treatments include topical steroids, intralesional steroid and phototherapy in the form of PUVA (psoralen & UVA phototherapy).

Question 31
Correct Answer: A

Urticaria is characterised by wheels or angioedema. It can be classified into acute (<6 weeks) or chronic (>6 weeks duration). Acute urticaria is a type one hypersensitivity reaction that is IgE mediated leading to degranulation of histamine from basophils. Causes may include, food allergy, drug allergy, wasp stings or contact to allergens. Infectious causes in the form of bacterial and viral infection have also been implicated.

The pathophysiology of chronic urticaria is less well understood. There appears to be a trigger which sets of an immunologic response to trigger histamine release. Chronic urticaria can be subdivided into the spontaneous form (i.e., idiopathic) or the physical urticarias. Triggers for physical urticaria include pressure, heat, cold, water, sunlight and cholinergic triggers such as exercise.

Question 32
Correct Answer: C

This is a classic presentation of Henoch-Schonlein Purpura (HSP). The diagnosis is usually clinical. HSP is a small vessel vasculitis which can affect other organs not just the skin. When faced with this presentation clinicians should always perform renal biochemistry and urine analysis to exclude renal involvement. If renal involvement is suspected, early discussion with the renal team is imperative to initiate further investigation such as a renal biopsy and initiate management.

Question 33
Correct Answer: B

The above is the correct histological description of psoriasis. Lichen planus is characterised by irregular epidermal hyperplasia forming a characteristic saw tooth appearance, with a band like lymphocytic infiltration obscuring the dermo-epidermal junction. Pemphigus vulgaris is characterised by intraepidermal blisters, and epidermal acantholysis. Bullous pemphigoid is characterised by subepidermal blisters and inflammatory infiltration with small eosinophilic abscesses.

Question 34
Correct Answer: A

The key in the question here is greater than 0.8 (i.e., 0.9 or above).
ABPI assessment:
0.9-1.2: Full graduated compression bandage (4 layer)
0.5-0.8: Reduced compression bandage

<0.5: wound debridement and care, referral to vascular surgeon.

Question 35
Correct Answer: C

This appearance is characteristic of impetigo which is a bacterial infection most commonly due to staphylococcus aureus. The correct answer is a bacterial swab. All the other options are unnecessary given no adverse features in the question. For more information on impetigo see answer to question 5.

Question 36
Correct Answer: A

A is the correct answer for bullous pemphigoid. B is the description for pemphigus vulgaris.

C fits with dermatitis herpetiformis. D fits with systemic lupus erythematosus (SLE). SLE also shows IgM, IgA and C3 bands which are also granular.

Question 37
Correct Answer: B

This is most likely a cold sore due to herpes simplex. The correct answer is viral swab taken from lesion fluid or vesicle fluid. The treatment for herpes simplex is aciclovir (topical or oral) which should be used as soon as symptoms start as it inhibits DNA polymerase of the virus inhibiting its proliferation. If recurrent, consider prophylactic aciclovir.

Question 38
Correct Answer: B

This autoimmune condition is caused by autoantibodies against desmoglein 3. This is a cadherin type epithelial cell adhesion molecule. Histologically, there is an **absent granular layer, and hyperproliferation of keratinocytes.** The result is easily ruptured superficial fluid filled blisters. It is most common among the Ashkenazi Jewish population.

Characteristics
- Mucosal involvement – usually the presenting complaint
- Easily ruptured, flaccid skin vesicles and bullae which are typically painful.
- Nikolsky's sign – extension of blisters upon slight pressure (direct Nikolsky) and sheering of epidermis on sliding pressure (indirect Nikolsky sign).
- Acantholysis on biopsy
- Immunofluorescence shows **IgG and C3 at the epidermis**

Management
- Corticosteroids
- Steroid sparing immune suppressive medications.

Question 39
Correct Answer: C

Contact allergic dermatitis is a delayed immune reaction (type 4 hypersensitivity) to a material. Typically, nickel can cause this. Patients typically have a delayed onset with redness, itching, and scaling. It is usually managed with potent topical steroids.
Contact irritant dermatitis is also a common cause of this presentation due to accumulation of soapy water under the ring if not washed off properly. However due to the presentation evolving over a few weeks, contact allergic dermatitis to nickel is more likely.

Question 40

Correct Answer: A

Contact irritant dermatitis is a non-allergic reaction to repeated exposure to weak acid or alkalis such as detergents. It can often be seen on the hands and presents as erythema and dryness; onset is usually acute. Crusting and vesicles are rare. Healthcare workers are particularly prone to developing this due to repeated handwashing.

Question 41
Correct Answer: B

The following patient has acute pancreatitis due to gallstones. Clues in the history include the 7F's: Fat, Fertile (contraceptive pill), Female, over Forty, Family history, Fair skin, and flatulent. The above describes Gray Turner's sign which is ecchymosis secondary to retroperitoneal haemorrhage. Cullen's sign is periumbilical ecchymosis.

Question 42
Correct Answer: B

Athlete's foot is a fungal infection named Trichophyton. This is also called tinea pedis. Appropriate first line measures include taking skin scrapings (often unnecessary) and treatment with topical terbinafine, miconazole or over the counter anti-fungal preparations. Nystatin is not an appropriate first line treatment for tinea. Nystatin is usually a first line treatment for candidiasis. Topical steroids should not be used unless tinea has been excluded as steroids mask the clinical appearance of fungal infections by reducing the symptoms of erythema and itching. This can lead to delayed diagnosis and treatment of tinea. Stopping the topical steroid subsequently causes a flare of the underlying infection.

Question 43
Correct Answer: B

Atopic dermatitis (eczema) is a chronic relapsing, remitting inflammatory skin condition characterised by dry, itchy, red rash typically seen in the flexural surfaces - such as elbows at the antecubital fossa and behind the knees. There is a genetic predisposition to atopic eczema linked to filaggrin protein which is crucial to epidermal barrier function.

Risk factors
- Irritants – soaps, shampoos, fragrances
- Infections of the skin such as staphylococcus aureus.
- Cold and hot climates
- Food allergy – more relevant in the paediatric group
- Pollen, dust mites, pet dander

Management
- Addressing provoking factors
- Avoid soaps and detergents
- Frequent application of emollients
- Topical steroids for flares
- Treatment of concurrent skin infection

Question 44
Correct Answer: D

This patient has contact dermatitis although the other differential to consider would be irritant dermatitis due to repeated wet work as part of her job. These have been described previously. Patch testing is the investigation of choice for contact allergic dermatitis. Various allergens are applied to the patient's back and assessed after 2 and 7 days respectively. Good hand care advice is essential to avoid irritant dermatitis.

Question 45
Correct Answer: A

Milia is a very common skin condition that occurs in half of newborns. They usually occur on the face and resolve within a few weeks.

Paper 4 Questions

1. A 60-year-old patient complains he has multiple bright red erythematous papular lesions on his torso. They cause no symptoms. On examination, they do not blanch with pressure.

What is the likely diagnosis?

A. Cherry haemangioma
B. Halo naevi
C. Spitz naevus
D. Port wine stain

2. A patient comes in with a red papule surrounded by capillaries on his chest. It blanches with pressure on examination. You diagnose a spider naevus.

Which of the following is not associated with spider naevi?

A. Liver disease
B. Combined contraceptive pill
C. Oral steroids
D. Pregnancy

3. A 52-year-old lady presents with dry, inflamed, thickened skin on her face, arms, legs and chest which is uncomfortable touch. She has returned from a holiday in Spain 2 weeks ago. She says this always flares up when she goes on a beach holiday and takes months to settle.

What is the likely diagnosis?

A. Sunburn
B. Contact irritant dermatitis
C. Chronic actinic dermatitis
D. Erythroderma

4. A 40-year-old lady complains of a raised firm lump on her shin that after initial growth, has remained the same size for years. On examination, you notice a firm 1cm pink nodule within the skin, not attached to deeper structures and indents on sideways pressure. She wanted it checked out as her friend has been recently diagnosed with skin cancer.

What is the likely diagnosis?

A.   Basal cell carcinoma
B.   Dermatofibroma
C.   Keratocanthoma
D.   Bowen's disease

5. A 70-year-old female presents complaining of confluent plaques of red to orange discolouration on her shins which can be painful. The skin feels hard and warm.

What is the likely diagnosis?

A.   Lipodermatosclerosis
B.   Acute cellulitis
C.   Deep vein thrombosis
D.   Erythema nodosum

6. A mother brings her 3-month-old infant to your clinic with a bright red lesion on his right upper eyelid. This lesion fades with pressure but gets larger when the baby is crying.

What is the likely diagnosis?

A.   Cherry haemangioma
B.   Cavernous haemangioma
C.   Capillary haemangioma
D.   Port wine stain

7. A 1-year old girl had flu symptoms – a high fever, sweating and shivery. A few days later she recovers, however develops a maculopapular rash over her body. On examination, she also has small red spots in her uvula and soft palate. She is currently feeling well.

What is the likely diagnosis?

A. Measles
B. Hand, foot, and mouth disease
C. Erythema infectiosum
D. Roseola infantum

8. A 16-year-old patient with a background of atopic eczema presents acutely with a painful monomorphic punched out rash which started on his face and spread across his torso over a few hours. He is feeling unwell and has a fever of 38.5.

What treatment should be started?

A. IV amoxicillin + metronidazole + gentamicin
B. IV methylprednisolone
C. Oral amoxicillin
D. IV Aciclovir

9. A baby is born with a deep red non blanching patch on the right side of the face, along V1 and V2 dermatomes. The lesion is unilateral and does not cross the midline.

Which of the following is associated with the condition above?

A. Sturge-Weber syndrome
B. Haemangioblastoma
C. Pheochromocytoma
D. Renal cell carcinoma

10. A boy presents with a fever and is irritable. A few days later he develops a maculopapular rash which starts behind the ears and then spreads to the rest of the body. On examination, you find Koplik spots in his buccal mucosa.

What is the likely diagnosis?

A. German Measles (Rubella)
B. Mumps
C. Measles

D.   Toxoplasmosis.

11. A boy presents with a fever and is irritable. He later develops earache and pain on chewing. You notice a unilateral enlargement of his right parotid gland.

What is the likely diagnosis?

A.   German measles (Rubella)
B.   Mumps
C.   Measles
D.   Toxoplasmosis.

12. A boy presents with a fever and is irritable. A few days later he develops a maculopapular rash which starts on his face and then spreads to the rest of the body. On examination, you find occipital and post auricular lymphadenopathy.

What is the likely diagnosis?

A.   German measles (Rubella)
B.   Mumps
C.   Measles
D.   Toxoplasmosis.

13. Which of the following statements about erythroderma is correct?

A.   Erythroderma is when specific conditions affect the majority of the skin
B.   Erythroderma is when 50% of the skin is affected by a generalised erythema
C.   Erythroderma is not caused by drug reactions
D.   Erythroderma is when 90% of the skin is affected by a generalised erythema

14. An 18-month-old girl is referred to your dermatology clinic with a recurrent history of small and large blisters and erosions to her hands, soles of feet, groin, buttock and knees. The blisters on the hands tend to occur when she is colouring with pencils. The areas on the groin and buttocks tend to occur after changing diapers. Her feet and knees are the worst affected. These tend to stay for prolonged periods of time.

What is the likely diagnosis?

A. Non accidental injury
B. Epidermolysis bullosa
C. Toxic epidermal necrolysis
D. Bullous pemphigoid

15. A 34-week pregnant lady complains of severe itching on her abdomen. On examination, you find a papular rash around her umbilicus which extends to her buttocks, thighs and arms.

What is the likely diagnosis?

A. Polymorphic eruption of pregnancy
B. Intrahepatic cholestasis of pregnancy
C. Pemphigoid gestationis
D. Dermatitis herpetiformis

16. A 34-week pregnant lady complains of severe itching on her abdomen. On examination, you find a vesicular rash around her umbilicus which extends to her buttocks, thighs and arms.

What is the likely diagnosis?

A. Polymorphic eruption of pregnancy
B. Intrahepatic cholestasis of pregnancy
C. Pemphigoid gestationis
D. Dermatitis herpetiformis

17. All of the following bacteria are found on the skin except?

A. Staphylococcus aureus
B. Escherichia coli

C. Staphylococcus epidermidis
D. Propionibacterium acnes

18. A patient presents with and multiple pustules on her hands and feet with associated fissures and thickened scaly, erythematous skin.

What is the likely diagnosis?

A. Palmoplantar pustulosis (PPP)
B. Chronic plaque psoriasis
C. Acute pompholyx
D. Keratoderma blennorrhagica

19. Which of the following conditions is associated with keratoderma blennorrhagica?

A. Reiter's disease
B. Behcet's disease
C. Inflammatory bowel disease
D. Psoriasis

20. A 38-year-old female is diagnosed with acanthosis nigricans.

Which of the following is not associated with this condition?

A. Lung cancer
B. Obesity
C. Diabetes mellitus
D. Acromegaly

21. Which of the following statements about albinism is incorrect?

A. Oculocutaneous albinism is inherited in an autosomal recessive fashion
B. Ocular albinism is inherited in an X-linked fashion
C. It is due to a mutation in tyrosinase gene coding for melanin
D. Albinism is due to the loss of functioning melanocytes

22. Which of the following statements about Merkel cell carcinoma is false?

A.　It is more common in patients with HIV
B.　It presents as a slowly growing solitary irregular red nodule
C.　It metastasises via lymph nodes
D.　Infection with a virus has been associated with a majority of cases

23. A female patient with severe acne vulgaris is started on isotretinoin.

Which of the following advice is the most important for this patient?

A. Contraception using oral combined contraceptive medication
B. Wear sunscreen during daytime
C. Avoid metronidazole
D. Do not drink alcohol

24. A penicillin allergic patient is admitted with sepsis from an unknown source and started on broad spectrum intravenous antibiotics. Minutes after commencement of the antibiotics, she develops flushing of her face, and an erythematous rash affecting her face, neck and upper torso.

Which of the following antibiotics is most likely responsible?

A. Clindamycin
B. Gentamicin
C. Vancomycin
D. Linezolid

25. Which of the following antibiotics causes Grey baby syndrome?

A. Chloramphenicol
B. Vancomycin
C. Clindamycin
D. Doxycycline

26. A gardener was cutting giant hogweed with a strimmer in a hot summer day. A few hours later, he began to develop red, itchy, painful hands. This later developed into inflamed oedematous hands with large bullae within the course of the day.

What is the likely diagnosis?

A. Phytophotodermatitis
B. Anaphylaxis
C. Allergic dermatitis
D. Contact irritant dermatitis

27. Which of the following viruses causes Orf lesions?

A. Molluscum contagiosum
B. Pox virus
C. Herpes simplex virus (HSV)
D. Human papilloma virus (HPV)

28. A 33-year-old male runner presents with extremely smelly feet. On examination, you find white clusters of punched out pits and macerations on the plantar surface of his feet.

What is the likely diagnosis?

A. Tine pedis
B. Pitted keratolysis
C. Erythrasma
D. Palmoplantar keratoderma

29. What is the likely diagnosis featured below?

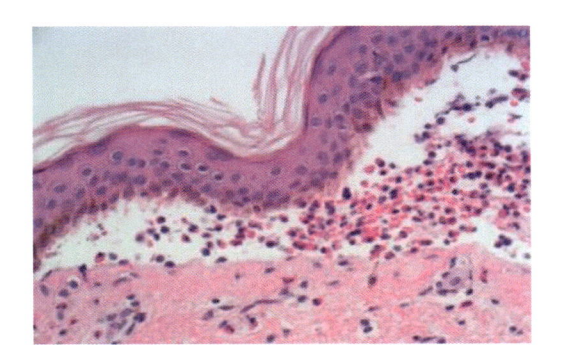

A. Psoriasis
B. Dermatitis
C. Lichen Planus
D. Bullous Pemphigoid

30. What is the likely diagnosis in the image below?

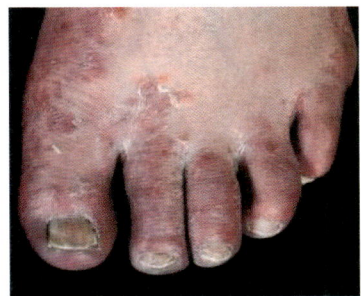

A. Tinea pedia
B. Pitted keratolysis
C. Erythrasma
D. Palmoplantar keratoderma

31. What is the likely spot diagnosis of this non blanching lesion below?

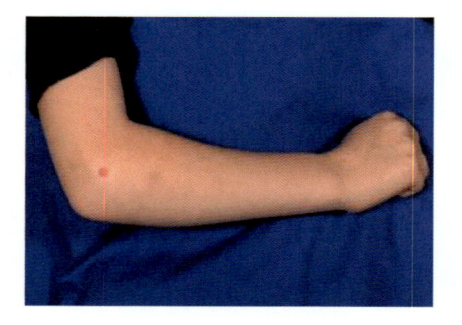

A. Cherry haemangioma
B. Halo naevi
C. Spitz naevus
D. Port wine stain

32. What is the likely diagnosis of this ulcerated painful area in the image?

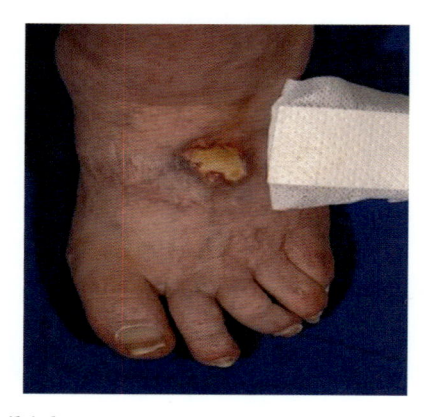

A. Pretibial myxoedema
B. Erythema nodosum
C. Pyoderma gangrenosum
D. Necrobiosis lipoidica

33. What is the likely diagnosis of the image below?

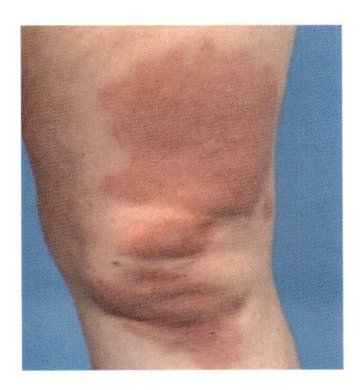

A. Dermatitis herpetiformis
B. Eczema
C. Idiopathic thrombocytopenia purpura
D. Plaque psoriasis

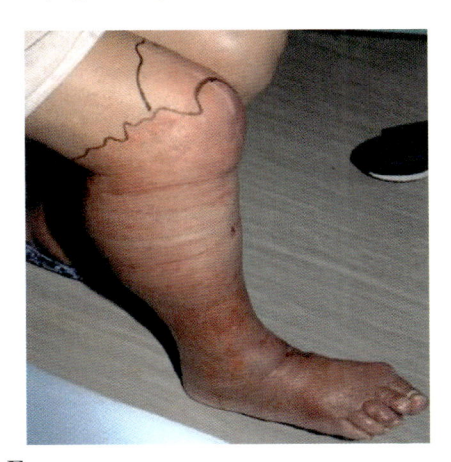

34. What is the likely spot diagnosis below?

A. Venous Eczema
B. Cellulitis
C. Necrotising fasciitis
D. Gas gangrene

35. What is the likely diagnosis below? The patient reports they are tender but there is no history of trauma. Similar areas are noted on the other leg.

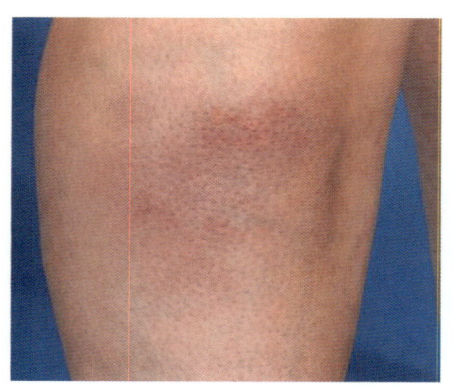

A. Pretibial myxoedema
B. Erythema nodosum
C. Pyoderma gangrenosum
D. Necrobiosis lipoidica

36. What is the likely diagnosis of this itchy rash on the hands of the patient?

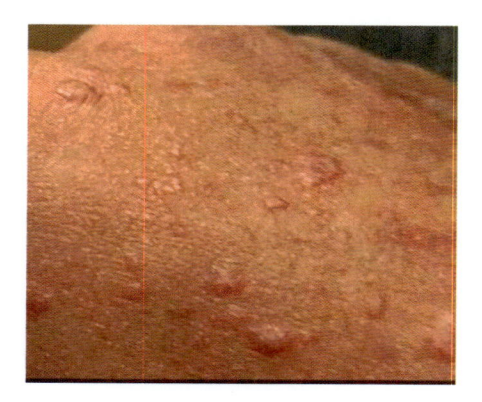

A. Lichen Planus
B. Discoid eczema
C. Guttate psoriasis
D. Dermatitis

37. What is the likely diagnosis below?

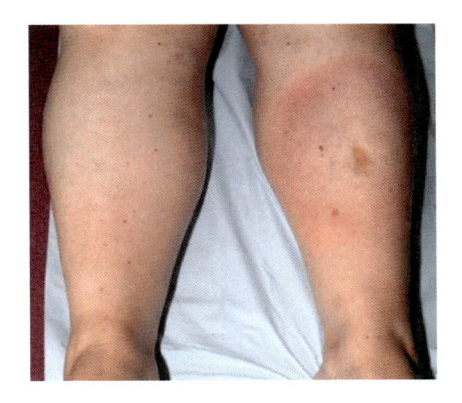

A. Erythema migrans
B. Erythema multiforme
C. Erythema nodosum
D. Pre-tibial myxoedema

38. What is the likely diagnosis of the lesion noted below?

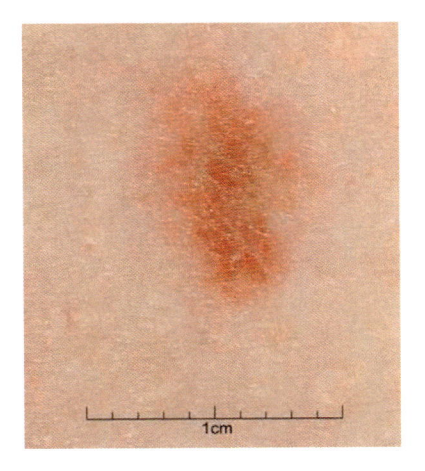

A. Bowen's disease
B. Melanocytic naevus
C. Mycosis fungoides
D. Squamous cell carcinoma

39. What is the likely diagnosis below?

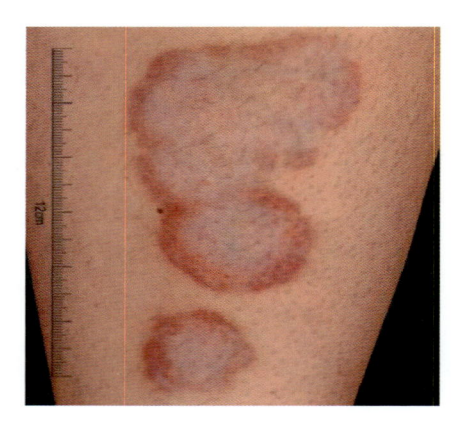

A. Necrobiosis lipoidica
B. Erythema multiform
C. Erythema nodosum
D. Pre-tibial myxoedema

40. This lady presents with multiple erythematous scaly lesions on the legs which are asymptomatic?

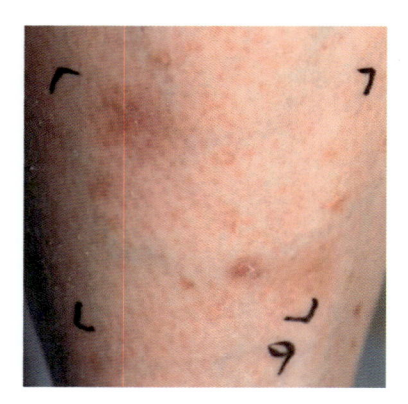

A. Malignant melanoma
B. Erythema nodosum
C. Pre-tibial myxoedema
D. Bowen's disease

41. What is the likely diagnosis below?

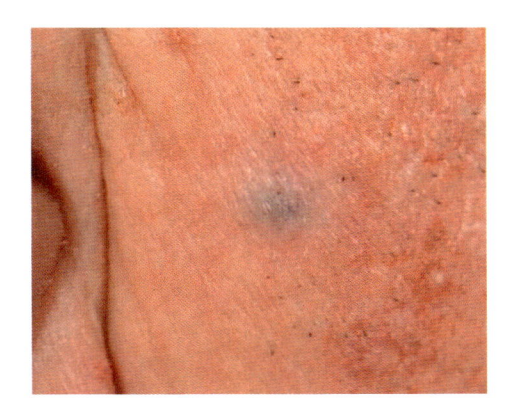

A. Blue naevus
B. Halo naevus
C. Spitz naevus
D. Port wine stain

42. What is the likely diagnosis of this scaly lesion on the forehead?

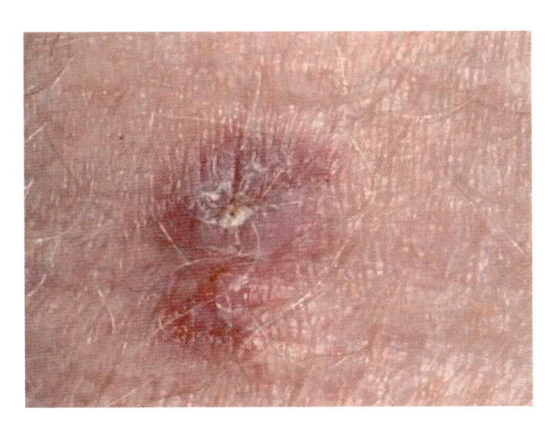

A. Ephelides
B. Actinic lentigo
C. Actinic keratosis
D. Seborrhoeic wart

43. What is the likely diagnosis below?

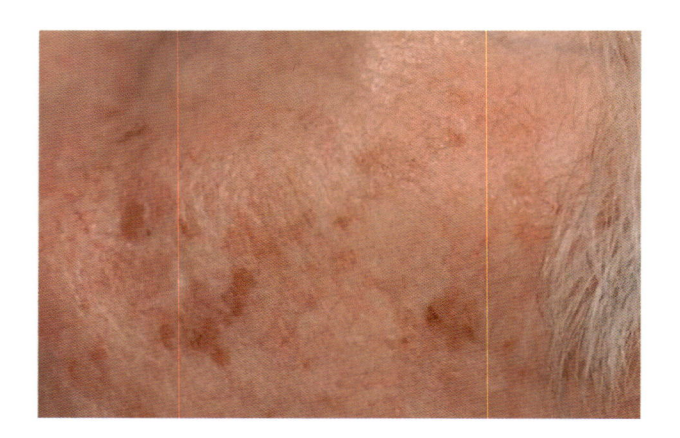

A. Ephelides
B. Actinic lentigines
C. Actinic keratosis
D. Seborrhoeic wart

44. What is the likely spot diagnosis below?

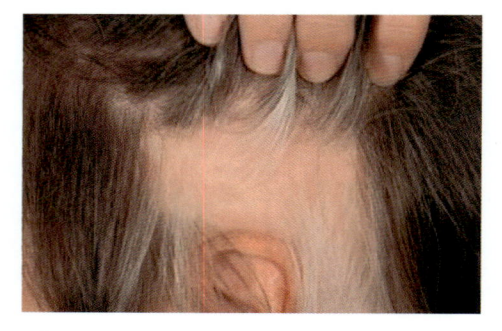

A. Anorexia nervosa
B. Fungal infection
C. Normal hair distribution
D. Alopecia areata

45. What is the likely diagnosis of this slowly growing lesion?

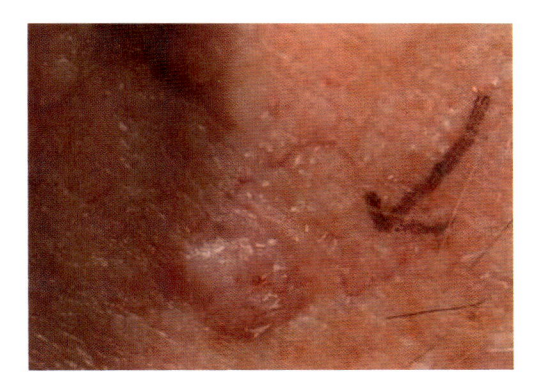

A. Squamous cell carcinoma
B. Basal cell carcinoma
C. Malignant melanoma
D. Basal cell papilloma

Paper 4 Answers

Question 1
Correct Answer: A

A cherry haemangioma presents as erythematous (bright red) papules which are typically non blanching and only very rarely found on mucosal surfaces. They are benign in nature. They are more common in elderly.

Halo naevi is a benign nevus with a white ring (halo) surrounding it. The inner dark nevus fades in colour to light brown and eventually to pink before disappearing. This is due to immunologic reaction to the pigment.

Spitz naevus is a benign melanocytic naevus that can be difficult to differentiate from a melanoma both clinically and histologically. It appears symmetrical, discrete smooth, firm papule. It can be pink, red-brown in colour. They usually occur in children and adolescents under 20 years of age. It usually grows over a few years.

Another interesting naevi is called a **Blue naevus** which occurs due to incomplete migration of melanocytes from the dermis. It can be macular, papular or plaque like, with a deep blueish colour, smooth surface and oval in shape.

Port wine stains are capillary vascular malformations which are present since birth and often occur in the face, often along the distribution of V1 and V2 dermatomes and never cross the midline. However, trunk or limbs may also be involved. They are usually red, non-blanching and grow as the child grows and develops.

Question 2
Correct Answer: C

Spider naevus is a red papule with surrounding capillaries which tends to blanch with pressure and can affect up to 10-15% of the population. Spider naevi can be idiopathic or associated with:
- liver disease
- pregnancy
- combined oral contraceptive pill

Question 3
Correct Answer: C

Chronic actinic dermatitis is a rare form of dermatitis of unknown aetiology, often called photosensitive dermatitis, provoked by UV radiation. It is characterised by pruritic, inflamed, dry skin which over years can become thickened. It occurs in sunlight exposed areas and more commonly in patients over 50, often with underlying multiple other contact allergies. This is diagnosed with photo-testing and photo-patch testing in specialist photobiology departments.

Question 4

Correct Answer: B

A dermatofibroma is a benign fibrous lesion often found on the extremities (histiocytoma). It is common in females and usually presents in adulthood and often related to old insect bites or minor trauma. Although it typically presents as a solitary firm papule or nodule on a limb, patients may have more than one lesion. Size can vary with up to 1.5cm lesions reported. They are firm and hard on examination, and when pressed side to side, have a 'pinch sign' which is indentation or dimpling of the lesion due to its fibrous nature - it is not tethered to the deeper tissue.
These lesions vary in colour from pink to light brown and often cause confusion with other sinister skin cancers such as a basal cell carcinoma. Patients are usually reassured that these lesions are benign.

Question 5
Correct Answer: A

Cellulitis is almost never bilateral and usually presents with associated symptoms such as a fever. Venous eczema is a form of eczema which occurs in either or both legs due to venous insufficiency. Associations include: venous leg ulcer; varicose veins; deep vein thrombosis; and cellulitis. Patients with underlying venous insufficiency are prone to developing areas of subcutaneous fibrosis and hardening of skin on the lower legs, often most common over the pretibial area or above the medial malleoli. These may feel swollen, itchy and associated with an aching pain. It may affect only one leg but is often bilateral. Chronic subcutaneous fibrosis results in an 'inverted champagne bottle' appearance with significant narrowing of the lower distal limb.
It is common in middle aged or older individuals with underlying venous insufficiency.

Other co-existing features:

- Discrete or confluent patches of deep pink to orange, brown pigmentation due to haemosiderin deposition.
- Atrophie blanche: white irregular scars with surrounding red dots

- Itchy, red, inflamed skin in acute phase, inverted champagne bottle appearance and hyperpigmentation in chronic cases.

- Venous ulcers

Question 6
Correct Answer: C

Capillary haemangioma is the most common benign orbital tumour in children. There are two forms, a superficial plaque type or deep. Capillary haemangiomas present early (2 months - 1 year). They are unilateral, asymmetric bright red lesions on the upper eyelid that blanch with pressure but increase in size with valsalva (crying). They may obscure the visual axis causing amblyopia. These grow within the first few months of life and then involute usually from 18 months onwards. Complete involution may take 3-10 years. Haemangiomas growing near important structures, or those which become ulcerated or painful due to rapid growth are managed with topical or oral propranolol - the treatment of choice. For stable lesions in older children, vascular laser may be used.

Question 7
Correct Answer: D

Roseola infantum (6th disease) is caused by Human Herpes Virus 6 (HHV6). It presents in infanthood (ages 6 months - 2 years) with a high fever lasting 3-5 days, cough, diarrhoea followed by an exanthematous rash with reddish pink papules which blanch, once the fever settles. This can be remembered by the 'rainbow after the storm'. It affects the trunk predominantly and usually avoids the face. A similar exanthem is seen in the soft palate and uvula called Nagayama spots.

Question 8
Correct Answer: D

This patient has eczema herpeticum which is a severe skin infection caused by herpes simplex 1 or 2. It is more common in children with a background of atopic dermatitis and presents with a rapidly progressive monomorphic vesicular rash as described above. This is a potentially life-threatening infection and should be diagnosed and treated promptly with IV aciclovir in hospital.

Question 9
Correct Answer: A

The above is a port wine stain (PWS) which is a vascular birthmark. It is usually ipsilateral, never crosses the midline and respects one or more of the trigeminal dermatomes. The lesions are deep red or purple and non-blanching. PWSs are usually idiopathic but can be associated with Sturge Weber syndrome which is a syndrome where the PWS affects the V1 and V2 distribution of the trigeminal nerve, as well as leptomeningeal vascular malformations in the brain and hence can present with seizures or even cause congenital glaucoma. PWS in Sturge-Weber syndrome may present bilaterally. The other options are associated with Von Hippel Lindau syndrome.

Question 10
Correct Answer: C

Measles is an RNA paramyxovirus spread via droplets. It has an incubation period of 10-14 days. Measles presents with a prodrome of fever, conjunctivitis and irritability followed by appearance of Koplik spots (white spots on buccal mucosa) which is pathognomonic, followed by appearance of maculopapular rash which starts behind the ears and spreads down the body.

Question 11
Correct Answer: B

Mumps is caused by an RNA paramyxovirus which spreads by droplets. It has an incubation period of 14-21 days. Mumps is usually infective 7 days before and 9 days after the parotid swelling develops. Symptoms include fever, irritability, malaise, earache, painful chewing and parotid enlargement which is bilateral in 70% of cases. Serious complications of mumps include meningitis, encephalitis and orchitis which can occur in the absence of parotitis.

Question 12
Correct Answer: A

Rubella (German measles) is caused by togavirus. It has an incubation period of 14-21 days. Rubella presents with a prodrome of fever and irritability followed by a maculopapular rash which begins on the face and spreads to the body. Occipital and postauricular lymphadenopathy are typically found on examination. These patients can go on to develop encephalitis, myocarditis, and thrombocytopenia.

Question 13
Correct Answer: D

Erythroderma is a term used to describe widespread erythema of more than 90% of the skin. Common causes include eczema, psoriasis, drug reactions and cutaneous lymphoma among others.

Question 14
Correct Answer: B

Epidermolysis bullosa is a general term used to describe a rare group of inherited conditions - it results from defects in proteins in the skin concerned with adhesion - resulting in blister formation or erosions. These may be inherited as dominant or recessive genetic disorders. The diagnosis is based on the site of blister formation within the skin.

It can affect the skin, mucosal membranes, gastrointestinal, and respiratory systems. The spectrum of severity can range from mild to severe disease which maybe life threatening. Key to diagnosis is recurrent history of poorly healing blisters and erosions which may arise spontaneously or following minimal trauma. This can present at or soon after birth or later on in childhood. There is may be a positive family history. There are four types:

1. Epidermolysis bullosa simplex: blistering within the epidermis
2. Junctional epidermolysis bullosa: blistering at the lamina lucida within the basement membrane
3. Dystrophic epidermolysis bullosa: blistering within the lamina densa of the dermis.
4. Kindler syndrome: blistering at multiple levels within and deep to the basement
membrane.

Question 15
Correct Answer: A

Polymorphic eruption of pregnancy is an idiopathic pruritic **papular** rash which occurs around the umbilicus, breast, buttock and thighs in the third trimester of pregnancy. It typically involves stretch marks and does not recur in subsequent pregnancies. It is treated with emollients and topical steroids.

Question 16
Correct Answer: C

Pemphigoid gestationis is an autoimmune condition which occurs in the second or third trimester of pregnancy with auto antibodies targeting the basement membrane proteins between the epidermis and dermis resulting in blisters. It presents with a pruritic **vesicular / blistering** rash around the umbilicus, buttocks, thighs and back.

The umbilicus itself is usually spared. Treatment is with oral steroids and antihistamine, it usually resolves spontaneously after delivery, however there may be a post-delivery flare up. It may recur in subsequent pregnancies and the patient needs to be made aware of this.

Question 17
Correct Answer: B

Staph. Aureus and epidermidis are common aerobic bacteria found superficially on the skin. They are the most likely causative organism in a patient with cellulitis.

Propionibacterium acne is an anaerobic bacterium found deeper within the skin, hair follicles and sweat glands. It is responsible for acne vulgaris. E. coli is a gram negative bacteria found in the gastrointestinal and urinary tracts and is responsible for urinary tract, gastrointestinal and biliary infections.

Question 18
Correct Answer: A

Palmoplantar pustulosis (PPP) is a chronic inflammatory skin condition. It is related to psoriasis but presents with characteristic multiple sterile pustules affecting the palms and soles of feet - with thickened fissures skin in these areas. It has a strong association with smoking. Other associations include other autoimmune conditions such as coeliac disease, diabetes and thyroid disease. Acute pompholyx is a form of eczema which occurs episodically with tiny vesicles or bullae formation in palms and soles.

Question 19
Correct Answer: A

Keratoderma blennorrhagica are thickened scaly patches with vesicular and pustular lesions on the hands and soles of feet associated with Reiter's disease.

Question 20
Correct Answer: A

This is a skin condition characterised by hyperpigmentation and hyperkeratosis of skin folds, particularly, in the axillae, groin, and posterior aspect of the neck. It is associated with obesity, type 2 diabetes mellitus, Cushing syndrome, hypothyroidism, acromegaly, and polycystic ovarian syndrome.
Gastric adenocarcinomas have also been associated with a variant of acanthosis nigricans, often called malignant acanthosis nigricans; it presents with marked hyperkeratosis and papillomatous velvety appearance. Lung malignancy has not been associated with acanthosis nigricans.

Question 21
Correct Answer: D

Albinism is a genetic condition which is most commonly inherited in an autosomal recessive fashion (oculocutaneous albinism). Ocular albinism, which is a rare form, is due to X-linked inheritance. Albinism is due to a mutation in the tyrosinase gene which results in the absence of melanin by melanocytes. Loss of functioning melanocytes results in loss of pigment in the skin and increased sensitivity to sunlight.

Question 22
Correct Answer: B

Merkel cell carcinoma is an aggressive neuroendocrine tumour which presents as a rapidly growing red nodule in sun exposed areas. It is more common in older aged men with immunodeficiency states such as HIV, organ transplant recipients or on drugs such as azathioprine.
80% of patients are found to have Merkel cell polyomavirus (MCPyV) which is believed to cause gene mutations. Spread is via the lymphatics system.

Question 23
Correct Answer: A

Isotretinoin is teratogenic and therefore, the most important advice is to remain on a reliable and consistent contraceptive whilst on the medication. This should be continued for a period of 4 weeks after stopping isotretinoin as it remains in the system for that duration of time.

Question 24
Correct Answer: C

This patient developed 'Red-man syndrome' secondary to vancomycin. This is a hypersensitivity reaction which occurs after rapid infusion of the antibiotic. It has also been reported to be associated with ciprofloxacin, rifampicin, amphotericin B and teicoplanin.

Question 25
Correct Answer: A

Grey baby syndrome is caused by accumulation of chloramphenicol antibiotic if used in newborns, especially premature babies. Doxycycline is also advised against use in children as it causes yellow, grey to brown discoloration of the teeth.

Question 26
Correct Answer: A

Phytophotodermatitis is a phototoxic reaction caused when a photosensitising agent in the sap from certain plants, interacts with ultraviolet A light from the sun. The Umbelliferae family, such as giant hogweed is commonly associated. It presents as vesicles or bullae which may have a streaking pattern and tend to settle in a few days. The hyperpigmentation may last a few weeks. This is not an allergic or hypersensitivity reaction.

Question 27
Correct Answer: B

Orf is a viral infection caused by sheep and goats. It is caused by a pox virus and appears most commonly on fingers, hands, or the face. It appears as a solitary, hard, reddish nodule which enlarges to form a blood-filled pustule. It is a self-limiting infection and tends to settle completely in 6-8 weeks, however, superadded bacterial infection is not uncommon.

Question 28
Correct Answer: B

Pitted keratolysis is a superficial bacterial infection affecting the soles of the feet, and less commonly can affect the palms. Multiple bacteria are involved, such as corynebacteria, *Dermatophilus congolensis*, *Kytococcus sedentarius*, actinomyces and streptomyces. It presents with smelling feet caused by sulphur produced by the bacteria and characteristic pitted and macerated clusters on plantar skin. This is more common in runners and farmers.

Question 29
Correct Answer: D

This is a histopathology slide of bullous pemphigoid, showing a clear cleft in keeping with a blister in the subepidermal plane and contains fibrin and large numbers of inflammatory cells including eosinophils.

Question 30
Correct Answer: A

There is widespread fungal infection affecting the skin of the dorsum foot and nails in this patient. The typical peripheral scale is evident at the edge of the erythematous rash. This typically starts in the web spaces but can spread if untreated and worsens with use of topical steroid.

Question 31
Correct Answer: C

Spitz naevi present as discrete smooth, firm papules or nodules commonly in children or young adults. They can be pink or red brown in colour.

Question 32
Correct Answer: C

Pyoderma gangrenosum is characterised by a red small papule that rapidly progresses into a very painful large necrotic ulcer. The periphery has a typical purplish undermined edge.

Question 33
Correct Answer: D

Discrete scaly erythematous patches on the extensor surface of the legs are characteristic of plaque psoriasis.

Question 34
Correct Answer: B

Unilateral erythematous leg with widespread oedema and evidence of pen marked at the periphery of erythema in this image, is typical of cellulitis.

Question 35
Correct Answer: B

Symmetrical tender nodules which are sometimes erythematous, characteristic of erythema nodosum.

Question 36
Correct Answer: A

Purple, pruritic, papules on the dorsal aspect of the hand is characteristic of lichen planus.

Question 37
Correct Answer: A

This is a bull's eye rash, also called erythema migrans, presenting as an extending ring of erythema, usually 7-14 days after the bite of an infected tick. This is a sign of Lyme's disease.

Question 38
Correct Answer: B

This is a pigmented lesion which exhibits a darker pigment and some irregularity of shape. It is called a melanocytic nevus; if ongoing change, it should be monitored.

Question 39
Correct Answer: A

Necrobiosis lipoidica appear as painless shiny yellow-red skin, typically on the shins with associated telangiectasia. Associated with diabetes.

Question 40
Correct Answer: D

Bowen's disease presents with slowly growing erythematous, hyperkeratotic patches or plaques with an irregular border. These are sharply demarcated, exhibit scaling with a pink or red surface and are often asymptomatic.

Question 41
Correct Answer: A

This is a macular lesion with a blueish colour, smooth surface and oval in shape. The correct answer is a blue naevus.

Question 42
Correct Answer: C

White, scaly plaque of variable thickness with surrounding redness; they are most notable for having a sandpaper-like texture. This is suggestive of actinic keratosis, common in sun exposed skin such as the forehead.

Question 43
Correct Answer: B

Actinic lentigines are benign areas of pigmented skin secondary to UV light exposure. They are the result of proliferation of melanocytes and accumulation of melanin within keratinocytes. They appear as flat, discrete patches of pigmented skin lesion on sun exposed areas. They are usually oval in shape and range in size from a few millimetres to several centimetres. They are differentiated from ephelides (freckles), as they do not darken following sunlight.

Question 44
Correct Answer: D

Alopecia areata presents most typically with patchy non-scarring hair loss. The re-grown hairs are initially white or grey as shown in this image.

Question 45
Correct Answer: B

This is an ulcerated pearly nodule with a pearly edge and associated telangiectasia. The correct answer is BCC.

Thank you

Thank you for purchasing the Dermatology Multiple Choice Questions and Notes. We greatly appreciate your support, and we hope that you learned vast amounts from this book.

If you are interested in finding more medical resources, follow us on:

Instagram: @bridgingthegapacademy
Facebook: @bridgingthegapacademy
Twitter: @bridgingacademy
Website: bridgingthegapacademy.com
YouTube: Bridging the Gap Academy

We are in the process of creating undergraduate and postgraduate courses, so please stay tuned.

Good luck in your studies!

Printed in Great Britain
by Amazon